CBD HEMP OIL

A SCIENTIFIC GUIDE FOR CBD USE AND PAIN RELIEF

MATTHEW STONE

© Copyright 2018 - All rights reserved.

The content contained within this book may not be reproduced, duplicated or transmitted without direct written permission from the author or the publisher.

Under no circumstances will any blame or legal responsibility be held against the publisher, or author, for any damages, reparation, or monetary loss due to the information contained within this book. Either directly or indirectly.

Legal Notice:

This book is copyright protected. This book is only for personal use. You cannot amend, distribute, sell, use, quote or paraphrase any part, or the content within this book, without the consent of the author or publisher.

Disclaimer Notice:

Please note the information contained within this document is for educational and entertainment purposes only. All effort has been executed to present accurate, up to date, and reliable, complete information. No warranties of any kind are declared or implied. Readers acknowledge that the author is not engaging in the rendering of legal, financial, medical or professional advice. The content within this book has been derived from various sources. Please consult a licensed professional before attempting any techniques outlined in this book.

By reading this document, the reader agrees that under no circumstances is the author responsible for any losses, direct or indirect, which are incurred as a result of the use of information contained within this document, including, but not limited to, — errors, omissions, or inaccuracies.

Table of Contents

Abstract	1
Introduction	3
Legal Status	9
Therapeutic Uses Of Cannabinoids	15
Everything You Need To Know About Cbd Oil	35
How To Use CBD Oil	44
CBD Should Not Be Mistaken For Thc As They Are Not The Same!	49
CBD Success Stories	66
References	77
About The Author	82

CBD Hemp Oil - A Scientific Guide For Cbd Use And Pain Relief

Abstract

Cannabis preparations have been used in medicine for thousands of years. However, concern over the dangers of abuse led to the banning of the medicinal use of marijuana in most countries in the 1930s. Only recently, marijuana and individual natural and synthetic cannabinoid receptor agonists and antagonists, as well as chemically related compounds, whose mechanism of action is still obscure, have come back to being considered of therapeutic value. However, their use is highly restricted. Despite the mild addiction to cannabis and the possible enhancement of addiction to other substances of abuse, when combined with cannabis, the therapeutic value of cannabinoids is too high to be put aside. Numerous diseases, such as anorexia, emesis, pain, inflammation, multiple sclerosis, neurodegenerative disorders (Parkinson's disease, Huntington's disease, Tourette's syndrome, Alzheimer's disease), epilepsy, glaucoma, osteoporosis, schizophrenia, cardiovascular disorders, cancer, obesity, and metabolic syndrome-related disorders, to name just a few, are being treated or have the potential to be treated by cannabinoid agonists/antagonists/cannabinoid-related compounds. In view of the very low toxicity and the generally benign side effects of this group of compounds, neglecting or denying their clinical potential is unacceptable - instead, we need to work on the development of more selective cannabinoid receptor agonists/antagonists and related compounds, as well as on novel drugs of this family with better selectivity, distribution patterns, and pharmacokinetics, and - in cases where it is impossible to separate the desired clinical action and the psychoactivity - just to monitor these side effects carefully.

Cannabis has been used in medicine for millennials. Investigations into the chemistry of Cannabis began in the mid-19th century, following a major trend in chemical research at the time, which centered on the quest for active natural products. Numerous alkaloids were isolated in pure form or partially characterized. Morphine, cocaine, strychnine, and many others were purified and used in medicine. However, most of the terpenoids - a major class of secondary plant metabolites, to which the plant cannabinoids also belong - were not isolated until the end of the century or even much later, and in many cases their purity was doubtful.

In 1840, Schlesinger was apparently the first investigator to obtain an active extract from the leaves and flowers of hemp. A few years later, Decourtive described the preparation of an ethanol extract that on evaporation of the solvent gave a dark resin, which he named "cannabin". It was, however, not until 1964 that $\Delta 9$-tetrahydrocannabinol ($\Delta 9$-THC), the major psychoactive component of Cannabis, was isolated in pure form and its structure was elucidated. Shortly thereafter it was synthesized and became widely available. These chemical advances led to an avalanche of publications on $\Delta 9$-THC, as well as on cannabidiol (CBD), a non-psychoactive plant cannabinoid. However, concern about the dangers of abuse led to the banning of marijuana and its constituents for medicinal use in United States and many other countries in the 1930s and 1940s. It took decades until cannabinoids came to be considered again as compounds of therapeutic value, and even now their uses are highly restricted. Here we present an overview of the addictive and side effects of cannabinoids versus their therapeutic potential.

CBD Hemp Oil - A Scientific Guide For Cbd Use And Pain Relief

INTRODUCTION

Cannabidiol, or CBD, was one of the first cannabinoids scientists discovered and is, today, one of the most researched compounds in the cannabis plant. We can summarize all that research into two simple points, the most important things to remember about CBD.

Cannabidiol (CBD) is a naturally occurring cannabinoid constituent of cannabis. It was discovered in 1940 and initially thought not to be pharmaceutically active. It is one of at least 113 cannabinoids identified in hemp plants, accounting for up to 40% of the plant's extract.

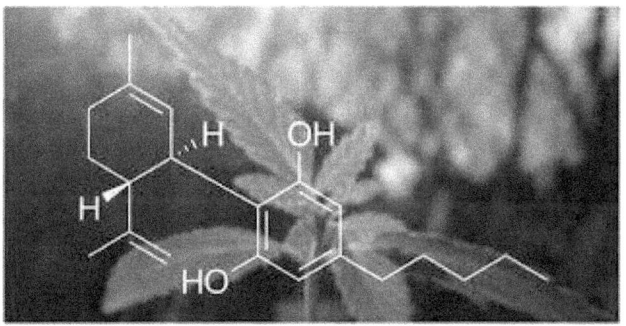

Formula - $C_{21}H_{30}O_2$, Molar mass - 314.464 g/mol, Melting point - 66 °C (151 °F).

CBD can be taken into the body in multiple different ways, including by inhalation of cannabis smoke or vapor, as an aerosol spray into the cheek, and by mouth. It may be supplied as an oil containing only CBD as the active ingredient (no added THC or terpenes), a full-plant CBD-dominant hemp extract oil, capsules, dried cannabis, or as a prescription liquid solution.

CBD From Plant sources

Selective breeding of cannabis plants has expanded and diversified as commercial and therapeutic markets develop. Some growers in the U.S. succeeded in lowering the proportion of CBD-to-THC to accommodate customers who preferred varietals that were more mind-altering due to the higher THC and lower CBD content. To meet the demands of medical cannabis users, growers have also developed more CBD-dominant strains. Cultural discussions and references to clinical studies that include CBD have influenced the demand for CBD-dominant products. Hemp is classified as any part of the cannabis plant containing no more than 0.3% THC in dry weight form (not liquid or extracted form).

What are the Effects of CBD? Does it Get You High?

You have probably heard of CBD in the news due to its wide range of medical applications – especially for children and adults suffering from chronic conditions. They clearly get relief from their ailments with the use of CBD, but the question everyone wants to know – are they getting high?

Does CBD Get You High?

No! CBD is 100% non-psychoactive, meaning it doesn't negatively impact your mind or mental process. In other words, CBD does not get you 'high' or stoned. There is no mental slowness or haziness caused by CBD – seriously, none.

You might be wondering how this is possible. It's because your association of cannabis is to the marijuana plants bread for high THC content – the specific cannabinoid that gets you high. However, cannabis contains many other cannabinoids – most of which do not get you high, like CBD. Some cannabis plants are bred for high CBD content exclusively – these plants are known as 'hemp' – and only contain trace amounts of THC (below 0.3% to be exact). The combination of high-CBD with extremely low amounts of THC is what makes the products derived from hemp plants non-psychoactive.

To reiterate, the cannabis plant contains multiple cannabinoids, however, only THC provides the traditional high associated with cannabis. CBD, the second most prevalent cannabinoid, is non-psychoactive and doesn't induce any 'high'.

What does CBD feel like?

Now you're probably wondering, if CBD is not going to get me 'high', then what is going to happen? Valid question. Without going too deep into the science, which you can do here, CBD affects multiple sets of receptors all throughout the body. Rather than binding to your cannabinoid receptors directly (like THC), CBD exhibits an indirect influence on these receptors, increasing the levels of endocannabinoids produced naturally by your body. For reference, endocannabinoids are produced naturally in the body and phytocannabinoids (like THC and CBD) come from plants.

The result is described by many as a wave of relief or relaxation that can be felt throughout the whole body when ingested orally or vaporized. Topical application result in a near instantaneous reduction in swelling, pain, and discomfort. To be clear, the effects are typically pretty mild, but that's the point – CBD targets the source of your problem while limiting symptoms – without interfering with day-to-day life.

Many first time CBD consumers look down at their watch 30 minutes after ingesting tinctures and think, "I don't feel anything, is it even working?" An hour later, they totally forgot about their anxiety, pain, inflammation – you name it. This example serves to illustrate the subtle, yet extremely effective healing properties of CBD. You won't feel anything out of the ordinary, but after 90 minutes you'll suddenly realize that you pain has totally melted away.

You may feel: Relieved, Calm, Relaxed, Pain-free, Comfortable, 'Normal', 'Better'.

We realize that some of these positive feelings are hard to quantify – but that's kind of the point – your body's endocannabinoid system serves to maintain equilibrium, or homeostasis, in the body. In laymen's terms this means its function is to fix what is wrong with you if you are ill and optimize your health if you are already well.

The Chemistry of CBD - How CBD Works

Have you ever wondered if the second most recognizable cannabinoid, cannabidiol (CBD) will also get you high.

In short, the answer is no, but surely you would like to know why!

All cannabinoids, including CBD, produce effects in the body by attaching to certain receptors.

The human body produces certain cannabinoids on its own. It also has two receptors for cannabinoids, called the CB1 receptors and CB2 receptors. CB1 receptors are located throughout the body, but many are in the brain.

The CB1 receptors in the brain deal with coordination and movement, pain, emotions, and mood, thinking, appetite, and memories, among other factors. THC attaches to these receptors.

CB2 receptors are more common in the immune system. They affect inflammation and pain.

Researchers once believed that CBD attached to these CB2 receptors, but it now appears that CBD does not attach directly to either receptor. Instead, it seems to direct the body to use more of its own cannabinoids.

Often when we crack open a cold bag of buds, we take for granted that we are about to perform a chemistry experiment. Every minute detail of the structure of THC—from how it behaves around water (hydrophobicity), to its electrostatics (distribution of positive and negative charges)—determines how tightly it will bind to its target, CB-1.

Though there are minor differences between THC and CBD, the later's bond with CB-1 is remarkably looser than it's cousin, THC, by 3-5 fold.

Despite minor stylistic differences, the only true chemical differences are in the highlighted regions. This break in the ring structure from THC to CBD allows CBD more flexibility, and the additional hydrogen (H) on the oxygen (O) allows for an additional type of bond (hydrogen bond). The additional hydrogen bond, and addition of the double bond are examples of differences in charge distribution, as discussed above.

You might think that despite its weaker attraction to CB-1, CBD would still cause a similar effect as it is still moderately bound, but you'd be mistaken. In fact, CBD is observed to have an opposite effect on CB-1 than THC.

There are a few perspectives that we must observe to get even a sliver of the story. Biochemistry does a stupendous job of being exceedingly complex!

The first perspective comes from the structure of CBD, which, as stated previously, is different from THC in its specific shape and distribution of charge. These differences, no matter how minute, can have drastically different effects on CB-1.

Now, let us look at the perspective of the receptor itself.

You may recall CB-1, a structure which was only recently determined, belongs to a class of receptor/signaling proteins known as

G-protein coupled receptors (GPCRs). There are entire textbooks dedicated to these proteins, so I will give you the quick and dirty.

The helices that permeate through the cellular membrane are very dynamic, and their movements are determined by the molecule that binds to it (i.e. THC or CBD), and they are extremely sensitive.

Despite the striking similarities between THC and CBD, the differences are distinct enough to have differential effects on these sensitive helices; moving in such a way to elicit opposing effects. Though these effects may seem minor, this type a receptor results in large multiplicative signaling cascades within cells.

Remember how I said biochemistry is exceedingly complex? We only observed one interaction, setting aside the myriad of resulting chemical reactions inside the cell. Furthermore, differences in how they affect our consciousness occur on a larger scale—more biology than chemistry if you will!

Though these atomic interactions are seemingly insignificant, they cannot be taken for granted when observing biology. After all, biology is an intimate, intricate, intertwining of physics, mathematics and of course, chemistry.

LEGAL STATUS

Cannabis is legal for either medicinal or recreational use in some American states. Other states have approved the use of CBD oil as a hemp product but not the general use of medical marijuana.

Some state and federal laws differ, and current marijuana and CBD legislation in the U.S. can be confusing, even in states where marijuana is legal.

There is an ever-changing number of states that do not necessarily consider marijuana to be legal but have laws directly related to CBD oil. The following information is accurate as of May 8, 2018, but the laws change frequently.

However, state legislators generally approve the use of CBD oil at various concentrations to treat a range of epileptic conditions. A full list of states that have CBD-specific laws is available here.

Different states also require different levels of prescription to possess and use CBD oil. In Missouri, for example, a person can use CBD of a particular composition if they can show that three other treatment options have failed to treat their epilepsy.

Anyone considering CBD oil should speak with a local healthcare provider. They can provide information about safe CBD sources and local laws surrounding usage.

Also, research local state laws. Most states require a prescription.

Non-psychoactivity : CBD does not appear to have any psychoactive ("high") effects such as those caused by Δ9-THC in marijuana, but may have anti-anxiety and anti-psychotic effects. As the legal landscape and understanding about the differences in medical cannabinoids unfolds, it will be increasingly important to distinguish "medical marijuana" (with varying degrees of psychotropic effects and deficits in executive function) – from "medical CBD therapies" which would commonly present as having a reduced or non-psychoactive side effect profile.

Various breeds/strains of "medical marijuana" are found to have a significant variation in the ratios of CBD-to-THC and are known to contain other non-psychotropic cannabinoids. However it is only the amount of Δ9-THC that chemically gives a legal determination as to whether the plant material(s) used for the purposes of extracting CBD are considered hemp, or considered marijuana.

Any psychoactive marijuana, regardless of its CBD content, is derived from the flower (or bud) of the genus Cannabis. Non-psychoactive hemp (also commonly-termed industrial hemp), regardless of its CBD content, is any part of the cannabis plant, whether growing or not, containing a Δ-9 tetrahydrocannabinol concentration of no more than three-tenths of one percent (0.3%) on a dry weight basis. Certain standards are required for legal growing, cultivating and producing the hemp plant. The Colorado Industrial Hemp Program registers growers of industrial hemp and samples crops to verify that the THC concentration does not exceed 0.3% on a dry weight basis.

United Nations

Cannabidiol is not scheduled by the Convention on Psychotropic Substances.

United States

In the United States, cannabidiol is a Schedule I drug under the Controlled Substances Act. This means that production, distribution and possession of CBD is illegal under federal law. In 2016, the Drug Enforcement Administration added "marijuana extracts" to the list of Schedule I drugs, which it defined as "an extract containing one or more cannabinoids that has been derived from any plant of the genus Cannabis, other than the separated resin (whether crude or purified) obtained from the plant."Previously, CBD had simply been considered "marijuana", which is also a Schedule I drug. In June 2018, the FDA approved oral use of CBD as an anti-seizure drug in treating rare types of childhood epilepsy. This is a contradiction as Schedule 1 substances by definition have no accepted medical use.

A CNN program that featured Charlotte's Web cannabis in 2013 brought increased attention to the use of CBD in the treatment of seizure disorders. Since then, 16 states have passed laws to allow for the use of CBD products (not exceeding a specified concentration of THC) for the treatment of certain medical conditions. This is in addition to the 30 states that have passed comprehensive medical cannabis laws, which allow for the use of cannabis products with no restrictions on THC content. Of these 30 states, eight have legalized the use and sale of cannabis products without requirement for a doctor's recommendation.

Although most states restrict the use of CBD products to certain medical conditions, manufacturers of CBD claim their products are derived from industrial hemp, and therefore legal for anyone to use.[65] A number of these manufacturers ship CBD products to all 50 states, which the federal government has so far not intervened in. CBD is also openly sold in head shops, health food stores, chiropractor clinics, optometrist offices, doctors' offices and pharmacies in some states where such sales have not been explicitly legalized.

Australia

Prescription medicine (Schedule 4) for therapeutic use containing 2 per cent (2.0%) or less of other cannabinoids commonly found in cannabis (such as Δ9-THC). A schedule 4 drug under the SUSMP is Prescription Only Medicine, or Prescription Animal Remedy – Substances, the use or supply of which should be by or on the order of persons permitted by State or Territory legislation to prescribe and should be available from a pharmacist on prescription.

New Zealand

Cannabidiol is currently a class B1 controlled drug in New Zealand under the Misuse of Drugs Act. It is also a prescription medicine under the Medicines Act. In 2017 the rules were changed so that anyone wanting to use it could go to the Health Ministry for approval. Prior to this, the only way to obtain a prescription was to seek the personal approval of the Minister of Health.

Associate Health Minister Peter Dunne said restrictions would be removed, which means a doctor will now be able to prescribe cannabidiol to patients.

Canada

Cannabidiol is a Schedule II drug in Canada. As such, it is only available with a prescription.] It is available as a spray, called Sativex produced by GW Pharmaceuticals in the UK, for use in multiple sclerosis. The Canadian Government announced that October 17, 2018 is the date when marijuana can be consumed recreationally without criminal penalties] indicating that various cannabidiol products will be freely available to adult consumers.

Europe

Cannabidiol is listed in the EU Cosmetics Ingredient Database (CosIng). However, the listing of an ingredient, assigned with an INCI name, in CosIng does not mean it is to be used in cosmetic products nor approved for such use.

Cannabidiol is listed in the EU Novel Food Catalogue. This listing only applies to isolated or synthetic CBD, not to crude hemp extracts or tinctures naturally containing CBD.

The European Industrial Hemp Association has issued a position paper suggesting regulatory framework in EU.

Several industrial hemp varieties can be legally cultivated in western Europe. A variety such as "Fedora 17" has a cannabinoid profile consistently around 1% cannabidiol (CBD) with THC less than 0.1%.

Although the World Health Organization listed Cannabidiolum in a list of International Nonproprietary Names for Pharmaceutical Substances (INN) on 30 June 2016. French and Spanish versions wrongly mention agonist action of CBD on cannabinoid receptors while the English version says CBD is a cannabinoid receptor antagonist.

Sweden

CBD is classified as a medical product in Sweden.

United Kingdom

Cannabidiol, in an oral-mucosal spray formulation combined with delta-9-tetrahydrocannabinol, is a prescription product available for relief of severe spasticity due to multiple sclerosis (where other anti-spasmodics have not been effective).

As of 31 December 2016, products containing cannabidiol that are marketed for medical purposes are classed as medicines by the UK regulatory body, the Medicines and Healthcare products Regulatory

Agency (MHRA) and cannot be marketed without regulatory approval for the medical claims.

Switzerland

While THC remains illegal, CBD is not subject to the Swiss Narcotic Acts because this substance does not produce a comparable psychoactive effect.[81] Cannabis products containing less than 1% THC can be sold and purchased legally.

Where to buy: CBD From Ambary Gardens or Visit the CBD Help Guide

Therapeutic uses of cannabinoids

Obesity, anorexia, emesis

Cannabis has been known for centuries to increase appetite and food consumption. More recently this propensity of the drug was substantiated when the CB1 receptor was shown to have a role in central appetite control, peripheral metabolism, and body weight regulation. Genetic variants at CB1 coding gene CNR1 are associated with obesity-related phenotypes in men. In animals, CB1 receptor antagonism decreases motivation for palatable foods. Rimonabant administration caused suppression of the intake of a chocolate-flavored beverage over a 21-day treatment period, without any apparent development of tolerance. CB1 receptors were found to be preferentially involved in the reinforcing effects of sweet, as compared to a pure fat, reinforcer. Rimonabant selectively reduces sweet rather than regular food intake in primates, which suggests that rimonabant is more active on the hedonic rather than nutritive properties of diets.

Rimonabant leads to significant weight loss in obese human subjects. Treatment with rimonabant was also associated with beneficial effects on different metabolic parameters and cardiovascular risk factors linked with overweight. In clinical trials rimonabant was found to cause a significant mean weight loss, reduction in waist circumference, increase in HDL cholesterol, reduction in triglycerides, and increase in plasma adiponectin levels. Patients who were switched from the rimonabant treatment to placebo after a 1-year treatment regained weight, while those who continued to receive rimonabant maintained their weight loss and favorable changes in cardiometabolic risk factors. Rimonabant was shown to be safe and effective in treating the combined cardiovascular risk factors of smoking and obesity. It also diminishes insulin resistance, and reduces the prevalence of metabolic syndrome. Many of the metabolic effects, including adiponectin increase, occur beyond weight loss, suggesting a direct peripheral effect of rimonabant. Therapy with rimonabant is also associated with favorable changes in serum lipids and an improvement in glycemie control in type 2 diabetes. The activity of rimonabant in the management of obesity has been described in recent reviews. It has been approved for the treatment of obesity in the European Union, and is sold under the trade name Acomplia. Surprisingly, the US Food and Drug Administration has declined to approve rimonabant, primarily due to its slight potential to enhance anxiety and suicidal thoughts. The atmosphere of consternation of possible legal action due to side effects may have led to this decision.

The other side of the same coin is anorexia. While in obese populations weight loss is the main goal, in other populations, such as patients with cancer or AIDS, it is an immense problem. Dronabinol (synthetic THC, known as Marinol and approved for the treatment of nausea and vomiting in cancer and AIDS patients) is associated with consistent improvement in appetite. It was found to be safe and effective for anorexia associated with weight loss in patients with AIDS, and is associated with increased appetite, improvement in mood, and decreased nausea. In clinical trials, weight was stable in dronabinol patients, while placebo recipients lost weight. Dronabinol was found to be safe and effective for treatment of HIV wasting syndrome, as well as in patients with Alzheimer's disease and with advanced cancer. The possible mechanisms of these actions have been reviewed. Cannabinoids have a positive effect in controlling chemotherapy-related sickness. They are more effective antiemetics than the dopamine receptor antagonists such as chlorpromazinetype drugs. Direct comparisons with serotonin (5-HT)3 antagonists, which are widely used as antiemetics, have not been reported. However, while these antagonists are not effective in delayed vomiting, THC is known to reduce this side effect of chemotherapy.

Pain

Cannabis has been used for millennia as a pain-relieving substance. Evidence suggests that cannabinoids may prove useful in pain modulation by inhibiting neuronal transmission in pain pathways. Considering the pronounced antinociceptive effects produced by cannabinoids, they were proposed to be a promising therapeutic approach for the clinical management of trigeminal neuralgia. THC, CBD, and CBD-dimethyl heptyl (DMH) were found to block the release of serotonin from platelets induced by plasma obtained from the patients during migraine attack. However, in other reports cannabinoids are much less successful in pain-relieving. In a clinical trial THC did not have any significant effect on ongoing and paroxysmal pain, allodynia, quality of life, anxiety/depression scores and functional impact of pain. These results do not support an overall benefit of THC in pain and quality of life in patients with refractory neuropathic pain. Similarly, in an additional clinical trial, no evidence was found of analgesic effect of orally administered THC in postoperative pain in humans. Other studies show much better results of pain relief. When THC was given to a patient with familial Mediterranean fever, with chronic relapsing pain and gastrointestinal inflammation, a highly significant reduction in pain was noted. Mild improvement was noted with cannabis-based medicines for treatment of chronic pain associated with brachial plexus root avulsion. In neuropathic pain patients, median spontaneous pain intensity was significantly lower on THC treatment than on placebo treatment, and median pain relief score (numerical rating scale) was higher. It was also effective in treating central pain. The administration of single oral doses of THC to patients with cancer pain demonstrated a mild analgesic effect. Patients who suffer from pain also tend to self-medicate with marijuana. In an anonymous cross-sectional survey, 72 (35 %) of chronic noncancer pain patients reported having used cannabis for relieving pain. Cannabis-treated AIDS patients reported improved appetite, muscle pain, nausea, anxiety, nerve pain, depression, and paresthesia. Not only THC, but also other cannabinoids can potentially affect different types of pain. Nabilone is a synthetic cannabinoid approved for treatment of severe nausea and vomiting associated with cancer chemotherapy. In Canada, the United States, and the United Kingdom, nabilone is marketed as Cesamet. A significant decrease in disabling spasticity-related pain of patients with chronic upper motor neuron syndrome (UMNS) was found with nabilone. Another cannabinoid, ajulemic acid (AJA), was effective in reducing chronic neuropathic pain, although cannabinoid side effects (tiredness, dry mouth, limited power of concentration, dizziness, sweating) were noted. Cannabimimetic effects with ajulemic acid in rodents have also been recorded.

The combination of THC with the nonpsychotropic cannabis constituent CBD has a higher activity than THC alone. The CBD/THC buccal spray (Sativex) was found to be effective in treating neuropathic pain in multiple sclerosis (MS). Chronic neuropatic pain can also be treated with cannabis extracts containing THC, or CBD, or with Sativex. The latter also was effective in reducing sleep disturbances in these patients and was mostly well tolerated. Sativex is the first cannabis-based medicine to undergo conventional clinical development and be approved as a prescription drug. It is efficacious and well tolerated in the treatment of symptoms of multiple sclerosis, notably spasticity and neuropathic pain. Sativex has been approved for use in neuropathic pain due to multiple sclerosis in Canada.

Multiple sclerosis, neuroprotection, inflammation

Inflammation, autoimmune response, demyelination, and axonal damage are thought to participate in the pathogenesis of MS. Increasing evidence supports the idea of a beneficial effect of cannabinoid compounds for the treatment of this disease. In clinical trials, it has been shown that cannabis derivatives are active on the pain related to MS. However, this is not the only positive effect of cannabinoids in this disease. In rat experimental autoimmune encephalomyelitis (EAE), a laboratory model of MS, THC, given once after disease onset, significantly reduced maximal EAE score. Reduction in the inflammatory response in the brain and spinal cord was also noted in animals treated with dexanabinol (HU-211 a nonpsychoactive synthetic cannabinoid). In another trial in rats, all animals treated with placebo developed severe clinical EAE and more than 98 % died, while THC-treated animals had either no clinical signs or mild signs, with delayed onset with survival greater than 95 %. WIN-55,212-2, another synthetic cannabinoid, also was found to ameliorate the clinical signs of EAE and to diminish cell infiltration of the spinal cord, partially through CB2. Using a chronic model of MS in mice, it was shown that clinical signs and axonal damage in the spinal cord were reduced by the synthetic cannabinoid HU210. To more fully understand the involvement of the endocannabinoid system in MS, the status of cannabinoid CB1 and CB2 receptors and fatty acid amide hydrolase (FAAH) enzyme in brain tissue samples obtained from MS patients was investigated. Selective glial expression of cannabinoid CB1 and CB2 receptors and FAAH enzyme was found to be induced in MS. In mice with chronic relapsing experimental allergic encephalomyelitis (CREAE), a chronic model of MS that reproduces many of the pathological hallmarks of the human disease, a moderate decrease in the density of CB1 receptors in the caudate-putamen, globus pallidus, and cerebellum was found. These observations may explain the efficacy of cannabinoid agonists in improving motor symptoms (spasticity, tremor, ataxia) typical of MS in both humans and animal models. Spasticity is a common neurologic condition in patients with MS, stroke, cerebral palsy, or an injured spinal cord. Marijuana was suggested as treatment of muscle spasticity as early as the 1980s. In an experiment in mice, control of spasticity in a MS model was found to be mediated by CB1, but not by CB2, cannabinoid receptors. In clinical trials, patients treated with THC had significant improvement in ratings of spasticity compared to placebo. In one case report nabilone improved muscle spasms, nocturia, and general well-being. In another case report, the chronic motor handicaps of an MS patient acutely improved while he smoked a marijuana cigarette. THC significantly reduced spasticity by clinical measurement. Responses varied, but benefit was seen in patients with tonic spasms. At a progressive stage of illness, oral and rectal THC reduced the spasticity, rigidity, and pain, resulting in improved active and passive mobility. However, in other clinical trials, cannabinoids appeared to reduce tremor but were ineffective in spasticity. Moreover, in one trial marijuana smoking further impaired posture and balance in patients with spastic MS. The inconsistent effects noted might be due to dosedependency. Improved motor coordination was seen when patients with MS, seriously disabled with tremor and ataxia, were given oral THC. In another study, cannabis extract did not produce a functionally significant improvement in MS-associated tremor. Suppression of acquired pendular nystagmus (involuntary movement of the eyes) was seen in a patient with MS after smoking cannabis resin, but not after taking nabilone tablets or orally administered capsules containing cannabis oil. There are also findings suggestive of a clinical effect of cannabis on urge incontinence episodes in patients with MS. In the treatment of MS, as well as in pain reduction described earlier, there is a preferential effect of a THC+CBD combination (Sativex). A mixture of 2.5 mg THC and 0.9 mg cannabidiol (CBD) lowered spasm frequency and increased mobility, with tolerable side effects, in MS patients with persistent spasticity not responding to other drugs. Oromucosal sprays of Sativex significantly reduced spasticity scores in comparison with placebo. Long-term use of Sativex maintains its effect in those patients who perceive initial benefit. Zajicek et al originally reported that cannabinoids did not have a beneficial effect on spasticity; however, there was an objective improvement in mobility and some patients reported an improvement in pain. Later the same group also found positive effects on muscle spasticity with prolonged treatment.

The subject has been thoroughly reviewed.

MS is not the only disease state where the neuroprotective potential of cannabinoids can be seen. In animal experiments, 2 weeks after the application of 6-hydroxydopamine, a significant depletion of dopamine contents and a reduction in tyrosine hydroxylase activity in the lesioned striatum were noted, and were accompanied by a reduction in tyrosine hydroxylase-messenger ribonucleic acid (mRNA) levels in the substantia nigra. Daily administration of THC over 2 weeks produced a significant irreversible waning in the magnitude of these changes, which may be relevant in the treatment of Parkinson's disease The cannabinoids have a neuroprotective activity not only in vitro but also in vivo: HU-210, a potent synthetic analog of THC, increases survival of mouse cerebellar granule cells exposed to 6-hydroxydopamine. In a model of experimental stroke, rimonabant reduced infarct volume by approximately 40 %. Rimonabant exerted neuroprotection independently of its cannabinoid receptor-blocking effect. In clinical trials, dexanabinol-treated patients achieved significantly better intracranial pressure/cerebral perfusion pressure control without jeopardizing blood pressure. A trend toward faster and better neurologic outcome was also observed. However, in further experiments, dexanabinol was not found to be efficacious in the treatment of traumatic brain injury. A wide range of cannabinoids has been shown to help in pathologies affecting the central nervous system (CNS) and other diseases that are accompanied by chronic inflammation. In a rodent model of chronic brain inflammation produced by the infusion of lipopolysaccharide into the fourth ventricle of young rats, the cannabinoid agonist WIN-55212-2 reduced the number of LPS-activated microglia. Direct suppression of CNS autoimmune inflammation was seen by activation of CB1 receptors on neurons and CB2 receptors on autoreactive T cells.

Atherosclerosis is a chronic inflammatory disease, and is the primary cause of heart disease and stroke in Western countries. Oral treatment with a low dose of THC inhibits atherosclerosis progression in an apolipoprotein E knockout mouse model, through pleiotropic immunomodulatory effects on lymphoid and myeloid cells. Thus, THC may be a valuable target for treating atherosclerosis. N-palmitoyl-ethanolamine is an endogenous endocannabinoid-like compound. Its concentrations are significantly increased in three different inflammatory and neuropathic conditions. The enhanced levels may possibly be related to a protective local anti-inflammatory and analgesic action. CBD has been shown to exert potent anti-inflammatory and antioxidant effects. High-glucose-induced mitochondrial superoxide generation, NF-kappaB activation, nitrotyrosine formation, iNOS and adhesion molecules ICAM-1 and VCAM-1 expression, monocyte-endothelial adhesion, transendothelial migration of monocytes, and disruption of endothelial barrier function in human coronary artery endothelial cells (HCAECs) were attenuated by CBD pretreatment.

In experiments with obese vs lean rats, rimonabant was found to be a potent inhibitor of sensory hypersensitivity associated with CFA-induced arthritis in obese rats, in which the inflammatory reaction is more severe than in lean rats. It may thus have therapeutic potential in obesity-associated inflammatory diseases.

Parkinson's disease, Huntington's disease, Tourette's syndrome, Alzheimer's disease, epilepsy

Parkinson's disease (PD) is a chronic, progressive neurodegenerative disorder. The main pathological feature of PD is the degeneration of dopamine (DA)-containing neurons of the substantia nigra, which leads to severe DAergic denervation of the striatum. The irreversible loss of the DA-mediated control of striatal function leads to the typical motor symptoms observed in PD, ie, bradykinesia, tremor, and rigidity. It has been proposed that cannabinoids may have some beneficial effects in the treatment of PD. In animal experiments cannabinoids provide neuroprotection against 6-hydroxydopamine toxicity in vivo and in vitro.

The majority of PD patients undergoing levodopa therapy develop disabling motor complications (dyskinesias) within 10 years of treatment. Recent studies in animal models and in the clinic suggest that CB1 receptor antagonists could prove useful in the treatment of both parkinsonian symptoms and levodopa-induced dyskinesia, whereas CB1 receptor agonists could have value in reducing levodopa-induced dyskinesia. In the reserpinetreated rat model of PD, the dopamine D2 receptor agonist quinpirole caused a significant alleviation of the akinesia. This effect was significantly reduced by coinjection with the cannabinoid receptor agonist WIN 55,212-2. The simultaneous administration of the CB1 antagonist rimonabant with quinpirole and WIN 55,212-2 blocked the effect of WIN 55,212-2 on quinpirole-induced alleviation of akinesia. In animal experiments, chronic levodopa produced increasingly severe orolingual involuntary movements which were attenuated by WIN 55,212-2. This effect was also reversed by rimonabant. In other studies, rimonabant was found to possess some beneficial effects on motor inhibition typical of PD, at least in some doses. The injection of 0.1 mg/kg of rimonabant partially attenuated the hypokinesia shown by PD animals with no effects in control rats, whereas higher doses (0.5-1.0 mg/kg) were not effective. A nigrostriatal lesion by MPTP is associated with an increase in CB1 receptors in the basal ganglia in humans and nonhuman primates; this increase could be reversed by chronic levodopa therapy, which suggests that CB1 receptor blockade might be useful as an adjuvant for the treatment of parkinsonian motor symptoms. High endogenous cannabinoid levels are found in the cerebrospinal fluid of untreated PD patients. Administration of inhibitors of endocannabinoid degradation reduced parkinsonian motor deficits in vivo. Thus, both agonists and antagonists of CB receptors seem to help in some parkinsonian symptoms. In clinical trials, the cannabinoid receptor agonist nabilone significantly reduced levodopainduced dyskinesia in PD. THC improved motor control in a patient with musician's dystonia. In contrast to these findings, some studies find no effect of cannabinoids on PD: orally administered cannabis extract resulted in no objective or subjective improvement in either dyskinesias or parkinsonism, no significant reduction in dystonia following treatment with nabilone, and rimonabant could not improve parkinsonian motor disability However, an anonymous questionnaire sent to all patients attending the Prague Movement Disorder Centre revealed that 25 % of the respondents had taken cannabis and 45.9 % of these described some form of benefit. Thus cannabinoids seem to be able to treat at least some symptoms of neurological diseases.

Huntington's disease (HD) or Huntington's chorea ("chorea" meaning "dance" in Greek) is a disorder characterized by a distinctive choretic movement, progressive motor disturbances, dementia, and other cognitive deficits. Neuropathologically, HD is characterized by a degeneration of medium spiny striato-efferent γ-aminobutyric acid (GABA)ergic neurons and by an atrophy of the caudate nucleus. Advanced grades of HD showed an almost total loss of CB1 receptors and a further depletion of Dl receptors in the caudate nucleus, putamen, and globus pallidus internus, and an increase in GABAA receptor binding in the globus pallidus internus. Loss of cannabinoid receptors is also seen in the substantia nigra in HD. These findings suggest a possible therapeutic role of cannabinoid agonists in HD. Indeed, arvanil, a hybrid endocannabinoid and vanilloid compound, behaves as an antihyperkinetic agent in a rat model of HD generated by bilateral intrastriatal application of 3-nitropropionic acid (3-NP).162 The reduction in the increased ambulation exhibited by 3NP-lesioned rats in the open-field test caused by AM404 (anandamide's transport inhibitor, which also binds to vanilloid receptor 1) was reversed when the animals had been pretreated with capsazepine (VR1 antagonist), but not with SR141716A, thus suggesting a major role of VR1 receptors in the antihyperkinetic effects of AM404. However, both capsaicin (VR1 agonist) and CP55,940 (an CB1 agonist) had antihyperkinetic activity

Quinolinic acid (QA) is an excitotoxin which, when injected into the rat striatum, reproduces many features of HD by stimulating glutamate outflow. Perfusion with WIN 55,212-2 significantly and dose-dependently prevented the increase in extracellular glutamate induced by QA. Thus, the stimulation of CB1 receptors might lead to neuroprotective effects against excitotoxic striatal toxicity. In a clinical trial CBD was neither symptomatically effective nor toxic in neuroleptic-free HD patients.

Tourette syndrome (TS) is a complex inherited disorder of unknown etiology, characterized by multiple motor and vocal tics. Anecdotal reports have suggested that the use of cannabis might improve tics and behavioral problems in patients with TS. Indeed, THC reduced tics in TS patients, without causing acute and/or long-term cognitive deficits. In another clinical trial, where tic severity was assessed using a self-rating scale and examiner ratings, patients also rated the severity of associated behavioral disorders. There was a significant improvement of motor tics, vocal tics and obsessive-compulsive behavior after treatment with THC. There was a significant correlation between tic improvement and maximum 11-OH-THC plasma concentration, suggesting a possible role of this THC metabolite on the positive effect of THC. In another, longer clinical trial, THC was also found to be effective and safe in the treatment of tics. In view of the positive effect of CB1 agonists in the treatment of TS, CB1 gene mutations were investigated. However, TS was not found to be caused by mutations in the CNR1 gene.

Amyotrophic lateral sclerosis (ALS) is a fatal neurodegenerative disorder characterized by a selective loss of motor neurons in the spinal cord, brain stem, and motor cortex. Many effects of marijuana may be applicable to the management of ALS. These include analgesia, muscle relaxation, bronchodilation, saliva reduction, appetite stimulation, and sleep induction. In addition, its strong antioxidative and neuroprotective effects may prolong neuronal cell survival. Indeed, treatment of postsymptomatic, 90-day-old SOD1G93A mice (a model of ALS) with WIN 55,212-2, significantly delayed disease progression. Furthermore, genetic ablation of the FAAH enzyme, which results in raised levels of the endocannabinoid anandamide, prevented the appearance of disease signs in these mice. Surprisingly, elevation of cannabinoid levels with either WIN 55,212-2 or FAAH ablation had no effect on life span. Ablation of the CB1 receptor, in contrast, had no effect on disease onset in these mice, but significantly extended life span. Together these results show that cannabinoids have significant neuroprotective effects in this model of ALS, and suggest that these beneficial effects may be mediated by nonCB1 receptor mechanisms. THC was also found to delay the progression of disease. Treatment with AM1241, a CB2-selective agonist, was effective at slowing signs of disease progression, when administered after onset of signs in an ALS mouse model. Administration at the onset of tremors delayed motor impairment in treated mice when compared with vehicle controls; moreover, AM-1241 prolonged survival in these mice. In a survey among ALS patients, cannabis was reported to be moderately effective in reducing symptoms of appetite loss, depression, pain, spasticity, and drooling. Cannabinoids were also proposed to have a role in the treatment of Alzheimer's disease (AD). THC competitively inhibits acetylcholinesterase (AChE) and prevents AChE-induced amyloid beta-peptide (Abeta) aggregation, the key pathological marker of AD. THC treatment also decreased severity of disturbed behavior, and this effect persisted during the placebo period in patients who had received THC. Compared with baseline, THC led to a reduction in nocturnal motor activity These findings were corroborated by improvements in the Neuropsychiatrie Inventory total score, as well as in subscores for agitation, aberrant motor, and nighttime behaviors; no side effects were observed.

Studies on cannabinoid anticonvulsant activity began in 1975, when CBD, and four CBD derivatives, (CBD-aldehyde-diacetate, 6-oxo-CBD-diacetate, 6-hydroxy-CBD-tri-acetate and 9-hydroxy-CBD-triacetate) were shown to protect against maximal electroshock convulsions in mice, to potentiate pentobarbital sleeping-time and to reduce spontaneous motor activity. Later additional CBD analogs were shown to be active CBD was found to be an effective anticonvulsant with specificity more comparable to drugs clinically effective in major, but not in minor seizures. Furthermore, it appears that CBD enhances the anticonvulsant effects of drugs in major seizures and reduces their effects in minor seizures. Hence, CBD was suggested as a drug for the treatment of children with pharmacoresistant epilepsy. The application of the CB1 receptor antagonists SR141716A or AM251 to "epileptic" neurons caused the development of continuous epileptiform activity, resembling electrographic status epilepticus. The induction of status epilepticus-like activity by CB1 receptor antagonists was reversible and could be overcome by maximal concentrations of CB1 agonists. Arachidonyl-2'-chloroethylamide (ACEA), a highly selective cannabinoid CB1 receptor agonist, enhances the anticonvulsant action of valproate in a mouse maximal electroshock-induced seizure model. There are currently insufficient data to determine whether occasional or chronic marijuana use influences seizure frequency. In one case report, marijuana smoking was proposed to induce seizures. In another study, patients suffering from secondary generalized epilepsy with temporal focus treated with CBD remained almost free of convulsive crises throughout the experiment; other patients demonstrated partial improvement in their clinical condition.

Bipolar disorder, schizophrenia, post-traumatic stress disorder (PTSD), depression, anxiety, insomnia

Cannabis use is common in patients with bipolar disorder, and anecdotal reports suggest that some patients use marijuana to alleviate symptoms of both mania and depression. In a case report, one female patient found that cannabis curbed her manic rages; others described the use of cannabis as a supplement to lithium (allowing reduced consumption) or for relief of lithium's side effects.

The effect of cannabinoids on schizophrenia is controversial. Neuropsychological results in THC-intoxicated normal volunteers exhibit strong similarities with data acquired from patients suffering from productive schizophrenic psychoses, as regards disturbances in internal regulation of perceptual processes. In a recent study, it was found that anandamide levels are enhanced in firstepisode schizophrenic patients, and that THC downregulates anandamide signaling. This observation possibly means that THC lowers endogenous production of anandamide, which may actually be a defense mechanism - presumably comparable to the known observation that administration of corticosteroids blocks corticosteroid synthesis. Data from experimental-psychological tests show that personality changes generated by schizophrenia progression are comparable to psychopathological phenomenon due to cannabis intoxication. In another study, psychosis, which develops or recurs in the context of cannabis use, did not have a characteristic psychopathology or mode of onset. First-episode schizophrenic patients with long-term cannabis consumption were significantly younger at disease onset, mostly male, and suffered more often from paranoid schizophrenia (with a better prognosis) than those without cannabis consumption. However, a trend towards more insight and of fewer abusive or accusatory hallucinations was seen amongst cannabis users. This argues against a distinct schizophrenia-like psychosis caused by cannabis. Less avolition and fewer apathy symptoms were detected in patients with schizophrenia and cannabis abuse than in those with no abuse. In another clinical trial, the role of CB1 receptors in schizophrenia was studied by administration of CB1 antagonist to patients. The group receiving the CB1 antagonist did not differ from the group receiving placebo on any outcome measure.

CBD causes antipsychotic effects. It was found to be a safe and well-tolerated alternative treatment for schizophrenia.

Post traumatic stress disorder (PTSD) is a term for severe psychological consequences of exposure to, or confrontation with, stressful, highly traumatic events. Cannabinoids are believed to help in such cases. AM404-treated animals showed decreased shock-induced reinstatement of fear. In conditioned fear and Morris water maze experiments, FAAH (-/-) mice and mice treated with the FAAH inhibitor OL-135 did not display any memory impairment or motor disruption, but did exhibit a significant increase in the rate of extinction. SRI 41716 blocked the effects of OL-135, suggesting that endogenous anandamide plays a facilitator role in extinction through a CB1 receptor mechanism of action. In contrast, THC failed to affect extinction rates, suggesting that FAAH is a more effective target facilitating extinction than a direct-acting CB1 receptor agonist. Acutely, the absence of CB1 receptors reduces the neuroendocrine response and does not affect the behavioral response to moderate stress. However, upon repeated stress or acute severe stress, CB1 receptor deficiency causes persistent behavioral inhibition. Repeated bell stress seemed to cause a cumulative fear in CB1 receptor knockout mice. In self-reports of substance use among help-seeking veterans, PTSD diagnosis was significantly associated with marijuana use. These observations suggest that the endocannabinoid system can be modulated to enhance emotional learning, and that endocannabinoid modulators may be therapeutically useful as adjuncts for exposure-based psychotherapies, such as those used to treat PTSD and other anxiety disorders. CB1 receptor gene polymorphism is known to modify transcription of the gene. In patients with Parkinson's disease, the presence of two long alleles, with more than 16 repeated AAT trinucleotides in the CNR1 gene, was associated with a reduced prevalence of depression.

CBD, and some derivatives, were found to cause a selective anxiolytic effect in the elevated plus-maze, within a limited range of doses. A single dose of nabilone produced only mild improvement in anxiety; in a repeated-dose treatment a dramatic improvement in anxiety was noted in the nabilone group.

The effects of marijuana on human sleep patterns were noticed long ago. Reduced eye movement density was seen, with some tolerance developing to this effect. THC is sedative, while CBD has alerting properties as it increased awake activity and counteracted the residual sedative activity of THC.

Asthma, cardiovascular disorders, glaucoma

Asthma is a chronic disease of the respiratory system in which the airway occasionally constricts, becomes inflamed, and is lined with excessive amounts of mucus. In animal experiments, after methacholine-induced or exercise-induced bronchospasm, marijuana caused a prompt improvement of the bronchospasm and associated hyperinflation. In humans, habitual smoking of marijuana may cause mild, but significant, functional lung impairment; However, a mild and inconstant bronchodilatory action was found for THC In other clinical trials, smoking marijuana or ingesting THC were found to increase airway conduction. Other plant cannabinoids did not provide effective bronchodilation. The daily use of THC was not associated with clinical tolerance. THC administered in metered volumes by inhalation from an aerosol device to patients judged to be in a steady state, increased peak expiratory flow rate (PEFR) and forced expiratory volume in 1 second (FEV1) and produced bronchodilatation. In another study, salbutamol and THC significantly improved ventilatory function. Maximal bronchodilatation was achieved more rapidly with salbutamol, but at 1 hour both drugs were equally effective. No cardiovascular or mood disturbance was detected, and plasma total cannabinoids at 15 minutes were not detected by radioimmunoassay. The mode of action of THC differed from that of sympathomimetic drugs.

In another study, THC induced sympathetic stimulation and parasympathetic inhibition of cardiovascular control pathways. The peak heart rate rise after THC was attenuated by atropine and by propranolol, and nearly abolished by atropine-propranolol pretreatment. Acute THC significantly increased heart rate, shortened pre-ejection period (PEP) and prolonged left ventricular ejection time (LVETc) without any change in afterload; it enhanced cardiac performance. Partial inhibition of this effect was achieved with prior (β-adrenergic blockade. In contrast, following the smoking of one to three marijuana cigarettes, the heart rate rose, cardiac output rose, stroke volume, ejection fraction, PEP and LVET did not change; thus, in long-term heavy users of cannabis, marijuana has no significant effect on myocardial contractility independent of its effect on heart rate. Cardiovascular effects of acute THC administration included increased sympathetic and reduced parasympathetic tone; supine tachycardia and increased blood pressure with upright hypotension were observed. With repetitive dosing supine bradycardia and decreased blood pressure with tolerance to orthostatic hypotension were observed. Rimonabant attenuated the hypotensive effect of smoked marijuana in male smokers, suggesting a role for the CB1 receptor in cannabinoid hypotensive action.

A number of studies suggest that there is a correlative, but not necessarily causal, relationship between glaucoma and systemic hypertension. Ocular hypertension (OHT) refers to any situation in which intraocular pressure is higher than normal, and is the most important risk factor for glaucoma. THC, CBN, and nabilone were active in lowering intraocular pressure (IOP) in rabbits, while CBD was inactive. Certain derivatives of THC were more active in lowering IOP than the parent cannabinoid; some topically used soft analogs that have no systemic effects were also active in IOP reduction. The effect on IOP of 2-AG was biphasic (ie, an initial increase in IOP followed by a reduction). In contrast, noladin ether decreased IOP immediately after topical administration, and no initial IOP increase was observed. AM251 blocked the effect on IOP of noladin ether, but did not affect the action of 2-AG. Topical administration of anandamide and arachidonyl propionitrileamide decreased IOP; rimonabant antagonized the IOP reduction, suggesting that cannabinoids lower IOP through CB1 receptors. Significantly, higher levels of CB1 mRNA levels were found in the ciliary body than in the iris, retina, and choroid. CB2 mRNA was undetectable. This expression pattern supports a specific role for the CB1 receptor in controlling IOP. When delivered topically to cat eyes with osmotic minipumps, whole marijuana extract, THC and other plant cannabinoids reduced IOP, while cannabichromene was inactive. Ocular toxicity was seen after THC treatment, consisting of conjunctival erythema and chemosis as well as corneal opacification. Although these changes also occurred with marijuana extract, their intensity was much reduced. In contrast, no ocular toxicity was apparent during administration of plant cannabinoids other than THC. Marijuana smoking was shown to reduce IOP as early as 1971; the effect was later confirmed. The peak effect of THC on the central nervous system coincided well with the reduction in intraocular pressure induced by the drug; However, hypotonia outlasted euphoria. The results indicate that THC may have value as a hypotonizing ocular drug. The functional responses after THC inhalation in sitting normotensive and hypertensive patients included invariable increases in heart rate followed by substantial decreases in systolic pressure, diastolic pressure, and intraocular pressure. The intensity and duration of the arterial and ocular pressure responses to THC were greater in hypertensives than in normotensive patients; the changes in ocular pressure paralleled the changes in blood pressure in glaucoma patients. A single sublingual dose of THC, but not cannabidiol, reduced the IOP temporarily and was well tolerated by most patients.

Cancer

The antiproliferative action of cannabinoids on cancer cells was first noticed in the 1970s. Since then cannabinoids were found to act on various cancer cell lines, through various mechanisms. Cannabinoids were also found to be suppressors of angiogenesis and tumor invasion. Our knowledge on the anticancer activity of cannabinoids is rapidly expanding; hence only results of recent research on this topic are presented here. The cannabinoid agonists HU-210 and JWH-133 promoted glial differentiation in a CB receptor-dependent manner. Moreover, cannabinoid challenge decreased the efficiency of glioma stem-like cells to initiate glioma formation in vivo. The nonpsychoactive cannabidiol triggered caspase activation and oxidative stress in human glioma cells. Human melanomas express CB1 and CB2 cannabinoid receptors. Activation of these receptors decreased growth, proliferation, angiogenesis, and metastasis, and increased apoptosis, of melanomas in mice. THC, through activation of CB2 cannabinoid receptors, reduced human breast cancer cell proliferation by blocking the progression of the cell cycle and by inducing apoptosis. THC arrested cells in G2M via down regulation of Cdc2. Cannabinoids induced apoptosis of pancreatic tumor cells via stress protein p8 and endoplasmic reticulum stress-related genes. These effects were prevented by blockade of the CB2 cannabinoid receptor or by pharmacologic inhibition of ceramide synthesis de novo. THC-induced apoptosis in Jurkat leukemia T cells was found to be regulated by translocation of Bad to mitochondria. Exposure of leukemia cells to CBD led to CB2-mediated reduction in cell viability and induction in apoptosis (although CBD is considered not to bind to either CB1 or CB2 receptors). It is noteworthy that CBD exposure led to an increase in reactive oxygen species (ROS) production as well as an increase in the expression of the NAD(P)H oxidases Nox4 and p22(phox). Cannabinoid-induced apoptosis of human prostate cancer cells LNCaP proceeded through sustained activation of ERK1/2 leading to G1 cell cycle arrest. Rimonabant inhibited human breast cancer cell proliferation through a lipid raft-mediated mechanism. In a pilot phase I trial, nine patients with recurrent glioblastoma multiforme, that had previously failed standard therapy (surgery and radiotherapy) and had clear evidence of tumour progression, were administered THC intratumorally. THC inhibited tumor-cell proliferation in vitro, decreased tumor-cell Ki67 immunostaining and prolonged the survival time of two of the patients.

Many drugs used today can cause addiction and are misused and abused, for example opiates, cocaine, benzodiazepines, barbiturates, cholinergic agonists, ketamine, dopaminergic agonists, amphetamines, and others. Nevertheless they are still an important part of our pharmacopeia. Marijuana was used for centuries as a medicinal plant, but during the last century, because of its abuse and addictive potential it was taken out of clinical practice. Now, we believe that its constituents and related compounds should be brought back to clinical use. The reasons are: (i) the therapeutic potential of CB1 agonists is huge, as described in this review; (ii) for local action, topical CB1 agonists, or agonists that do not penetrate the blood-brain barrier, can be used; (iii) cannabinoids acting specifically on CB2 receptors, which cause no psychoactivity, may be used on peripheral targets (such as osteoporosis, which is only one of many examples); (iv) there are additional, new cannabinoid targets distinct from the CB1/CB2 receptors which do not cause psychoactivity; (v) there are cannabinoids, such as CBD, which do not cause psychoactivity, but have various therapeutic effects.

The endocannabinoid system is a very complex one and regulates numerous processes, in parallel with other wellknown systems, such as the adrenergic, cholinergic, and dopaminergic systems. Neglecting the potential clinical uses of such a system is, in our view, unacceptable; instead we need to work on more selective agonists/antagonists, more selective distribution patterns, and in cases where it is impossible to separate between the desired clinical action and the psychoactivity, to monitor these side effects carefully.

Everything you need to know about CBD oil

People take or apply cannabidiol to treat a variety of symptoms, but its use is controversial. There is some confusion about what it is and the effects it has on the human body.

Cannabidiol (CBD) may have some health benefits, and it may also pose risks. Products containing the compound are now legal in many American states where marijuana is not.

In June 2018, the United States of America Food and Drug Administration (FDA) approved the prescription use of Epidiolex, a purified form of CBD oil, for treating two types of epilepsy.

What is CBD oil?

CBD is one of many compounds, known as cannabinoids, in the cannabis plant. Researchers have been looking at the potential therapeutic uses of CBD.

Oils that contain concentrations of CBD are known as CBD oils. The concentrations and the uses of these oils vary.

Is CBD marijuana?

CBD oil is a cannabinoid derived from the cannabis plant.

Until recently, the best-known compound in cannabis was delta-9 tetrahydrocannabinol (THC). This is the most active ingredient in marijuana.

Marijuana contains both THC and CBD, and these compounds have different effects.

THC creates a mind-altering "high" when it is broken down by heat and introduced into the body. This results from smoking marijuana or using it in cooking, for example.

Unlike THC, CBD is not psychoactive. This means that it does not change the state of mind of the person who uses it.

However, CBD does appear to produce significant changes in the body, and some research suggests that it has medical benefits.

The least processed form of the cannabis plant, known as hemp, contains most of the CBD used medicinally. Though hemp and marijuana come from the same plant, Cannabis sativa, the two are very different.

Over the years, marijuana farmers have selectively bred their plants to contain high levels of THC and other compounds that interested them, often because the compounds produced a smell or had another effect on the plant's flowers.

However, hemp farmers have rarely modified the plant. These hemp plants are used to create CBD oil.

Benefits

Because of the way that CBD acts in the body, it has many potential benefits.

Natural pain relief and anti-inflammatory properties

People tend to use prescription or over-the-counter drugs to relieve stiffness and pain, including chronic pain.

Some people believe that CBD offers a more natural alternative.

Authors of a study published in the Journal of Experimental

Medicine found that CBD significantly reduced chronic inflammation and pain in some mice and rats.

The researchers suggested that the non-psychoactive compounds in marijuana, such as CBD, could constitute a new treatment for chronic pain.

Quitting smoking and drug withdrawals

Some promising evidence suggests that CBD use may help people to quit smoking. A pilot study published in Addictive Behaviors found that smokers who used inhalers containing CBD smoked fewer cigarettes than usual and had no further cravings for nicotine.

A similar review, published in Neurotherapeutics found that CBD may be a promising treatment for people with opioid addiction disorders.

The researchers noted that CBD reduced some symptoms associated with substance use disorders. These included anxiety, mood-related symptoms, pain, and insomnia.

More research is necessary, but these findings suggest that CBD may help to prevent or reduce withdrawal symptoms.

Epilepsy

After researching the safety and effectiveness of CBD oil for treating epilepsy, the FDA approved the use of CBD (Epidiolex) as a therapy for two rare conditions characterized by of epileptic seizures.

In the U.S., a doctor can prescribe Epidiolex to treat:

Lennox-Gastaut syndrome (LGS), a condition that appears between the ages of 3 and 5 years and involves different kinds of seizures.

Dravet syndrome (DS), a rare genetic condition that appears in the first year of life and involves frequent, fever-related seizures.

The types of seizures that characterize LGS or DS are difficult to control with other types of medication.

The FDA specified that doctors could not prescribe Epidiolex for children younger than 2 years. A physician or pharmacist will determine the right dosage based on body weight.

Other neurological symptoms and disorders

Researchers are studying the effects of CBD on various neuropsychiatric disorders.

Authors of a 2014 review noted that CBD has anti-seizure properties and a low risk of side effects for people with epilepsy.

Studies suggest that CBD may also treat many complications linked to epilepsy, such as neurodegeneration, neuronal injury, and psychiatric diseases.

Another study, published in Current Pharmaceutical Design, found that CBD may produce effects similar to those of certain antipsychotic drugs, and that the compound may provide a safe and effective treatment for people with schizophrenia.

Fighting cancer

Some researchers have found that CBD may prove to combat cancer.

Authors of a review published in the British Journal of Clinical Pharmacology found evidence that CBD significantly helped to prevent the spread of cancer.

In addition, the researchers noted that the compound tends to suppress the growth of cancer cells and promote their destruction.

The authors pointed out that CBD has low levels of toxicity and called for further research into its potential as an accompaniment to standard cancer treatments.

Anxiety disorders

Doctors often advise people with chronic anxiety to avoid cannabis, as THC can trigger or amplify feelings of anxiousness and paranoia.

However, authors of a review from Neurotherapeutics found that CBD may help to reduce anxiety in people with certain related disorders.

According to the review, CBD may reduce anxiety-related behaviors in people with conditions such as: post-traumatic stress disorder, general anxiety disorder, panic disorder, social anxiety disorder, obsessive-compulsive disorder.

The authors noted that current treatments for these disorders can lead to additional symptoms and side effects, which can cause some people to stop taking them.

No further definitive evidence currently links CBD to adverse effects, and the authors called for further studies of the compound as a treatment for anxiety.

Type 1 diabetes

Type 1 diabetes results from inflammation that occurs when the immune system attacks cells in the pancreas.

Research published in 2016 by Clinical Hemorheology and Microcirculation found that CBD may ease this inflammation in the pancreas. This may be the first step in finding a CBD-based treatment for type 1 diabetes.

A paper presented in the same year in Lisbon, Portugal, suggested that CBD may reduce inflammation and protect against or delay the development of type 1 diabetes.

Acne

Acne treatment is another promising use for CBD. The condition is caused, in part, by inflammation and overworked sebaceous glands in the body.

A 2014 study published by the Journal of Clinical Investigation found that CBD helps to lower the production of sebum that leads to acne, partly because of its anti-inflammatory effect on the body. Sebum is an oily substance, and overproduction can cause acne.

CBD could become a future treatment for acne vulgaris, the most common form of acne.

Alzheimer's disease

Initial research published in the Journal of Alzheimer's Disease found that CBD was able to prevent the development of social recognition deficit in participants.

This means that CBD could help people in the early stages of Alzheimer's to keep the ability to recognize the faces of people that they know.

This is the first evidence that CBD may slow the progression of Alzheimer's disease.

CBD oil for epilepsy

In June 2018, the FDA approved the use of CBD to treat two types of epilepsy.

Dr. Scott Gottlieb, writing for the FDA on 25 June, stated:

"Today, the FDA approved a purified form of the drug cannabidiol (CBD). This is one of more than 80 active chemicals in marijuana. The new product was approved to treat seizures associated with two rare, severe forms of epilepsy in patients two years of age and older."

Dr. Gottlieb is careful to point out that:

The FDA have not approved the use of marijuana or all of its components.

The association has only approved a purified version of one CBD medication, for a precise therapeutic purpose.

The decision to approve the product was based on the results of sound clinical trials.

Patients will receive the medication in a reliable dosages.

Side effects

Many small-scale studies have looked into the safety of CBD in adults. They concluded that adults tend to tolerate a wide range of doses well.

Researchers have found no significant side effects on the central nervous system, the vital signs, or mood, even among people who used high dosages.

The most common side effect was tiredness. Also, some people reported diarrhea and changes in appetite or weight.

Risks

There is still a lack of available long-term safety data.

Also, to date, researchers have not performed studies involving children.

Side effects of Epidiolex

Concerning the product that the FDA approved to treat two types of epilepsy, researchers noticed following adverse effects in clinical trials: liver problems, symptoms related to the central nervous system, such as irritability and lethargy, reduced appetite, gastrointestinal problems, infections, rashes and other sensitivity reactions, reduced urination, breathing problems.

The patient information leaflet notes that there is a risk of worsening depression or suicidal thoughts. It is important to monitor anyone who is using this drug for signs of mood change.

Research suggests that a person taking the product is unlikely to form a dependency.

Side effects of other uses of CBD

There is often a lack of evidence regarding the safety of new or alternative treatment options. Usually, researchers have not performed the full array of tests.

Anyone who is considering using CBD should talk to a qualified healthcare practitioner beforehand.

The FDA have only approved CBD for the treatment of two rare and severe forms of epilepsy.

When drugs do not have FDA approval, it can be difficult to know whether a product contains a safe or effective level of CBD. Unapproved products may not have the properties or contents stated on the packaging.

It is important to note that researchers have linked marijuana use during pregnancy to impairments in the fetal development of neurons. Regular use among teens is associated with issues concerning memory, behavior, and intelligence.

How to use CBD Oil

A person can use CBD oil in different ways to relieve various symptoms.

If a doctor prescribes it to treat LGS or DS, it is important to follow their instructions.

CBD-based products come in many forms. Some can be mixed into different foods or drinks or taken from a pipette or dropper.

Others are available in capsules or as a thick paste to be massaged into the skin. Some products are available as sprays to be administered under the tongue.

Recommended dosages vary between individuals, and depend on factors such as body weight, the concentration of the product, and the health issue.

Some people consider taking CBD oil to help treat: chronic pain, epilepsy, Parkinson's disease, Huntington's disease, sleep disorders, glaucoma.

Due to the lack of FDA regulation for most CBD products, seek advice from a medical professional before determining the best dosage.

As regulation in the U.S. increases, more specific dosages and prescriptions will start to emerge.

After discussing dosages and risks with a doctor, and researching regional local laws, it is important to compare different brands of CBD oil.

Several CBD oils with different applications are available to purchase online.

Q:

CBD has been tested and approved for one specific use. Does this mean it is safe and will soon have approval for other uses?

A:

The research is emerging to support the use of CBD for numerous conditions, as well as looking closely at safety, side effects, and long-term effects.

There are some valid concerns about long-term use that must be tested before CBD can be recommended for other diseases. As one approach to pain management, it is seen as an alternative option to the addicting narcotics.

The use of CBD oil might complement a medical approach to treating physical and mental diseases. It is worth discussing with your doctor.

Debra Rose Wilson, PhD, MSN, RN, IBCLC, AHN-BC, CHT

Answers represent the opinions of our medical experts. All content is strictly informational and should not be considered medical advice.

HOW-TO-USE-HEMP-OIL

You've made the decision to try CBD hemp oil in the liquid form of a tincture. Now you're likely wondering how to use hemp oil, or how to know if it's working for you.

We'll go over the following topics:

- Basics of using a tincture
- How to be safe when starting your hemp routine
- Shake, dispense, absorb, and repeat

- What to expect from your hemp oil
- Great hemp product recommendations
- How to find more information

Let's begin with the basics.

What is a Tincture? Tinctures are liquid extracts of plant or herbal materials, explicitly intended for oral (by mouth) use. Using them is extremely simple.

Thanks to the commonly used dropper top, you can easily measure an exact amount.

Educate yourself on the benefits of hemp oil and read about how other people are using it and determining how much to take. The manufacture recommended serving size on hemp supplements may not be perfect for everyone, so we encourage you to experiment.

If you receive a tincture and it's not sealed with either a plastic safety seal or a locked top, please contact the seller and request a new one. Many hemp-based herbal products on the market are made in small, niche facilities and are susceptible to human error. Be safe!

Step 1

Shake well!

Separation in hemp oil products is completely natural and to be expected. Some bottles are impossible to see into (which is good — dark bottles help block light for optimal shelf life), but if you can, take note of how the oil tends to settle onto the bottom. Once you start shaking, it quickly blends. I can't stress how important this step is. If you don't shake it, you'll likely end up consuming straight grape seed and coconut oil. It's not the tastiest experience, and won't be very beneficial for you either.

Step 2

Squeeze the dropper top to fill the pipette with oil and dispense the oil under your tongue. You can swish it around a little, but most people like to just let it sit (that way you avoid some of the hemp taste — albeit Tasty Drops actually tastes great if you choose a flavored version). You can add as many droppers full as needed; don't feel you need to restrict yourself to the recommended serving size. The phytocannabinoids in our proprietary blend are non-psychoactive. However, many people have noted a slight sedative effect at larger quantities. This may be beneficial if you have trouble sleeping, so consider using it before bed.

Allow the oil to absorb into your system by holding the oil in your mouth for 60-90 seconds before swallowing. You may choose to swish it around, but it's not necessary. If you find the flavor to be too strong, take a drink of juice as you ingest the oil to mask that hempy flavor (apple cider works very well).

Step 3

Repeat as necessary throughout the day. As mentioned above, hemp oil may be slightly sedative at higher amounts, or simply calming and relaxing at a lower serving size.

Results

Tasty Hemp Oil drops is a food supplement that can help support overall well-being. The natural constituents (called "phytocannabinoids") work by interacting with your Endocannabinoid System.

We recommend two weeks of consistent usage for the phytocannabinoids to build up in your system and for your body to understand what to do with it. If you feel it's not working for you after that time, try increasing your serving size. If that still doesn't help, email or call us for help.

CBD SHOULD NOT BE MISTAKEN FOR THC AS THEY ARE NOT THE SAME!

What then is THC (Tetrahydrocannabinol) And What Does It Do?

Here's everything you need to know about this chemical compound.

Throughout its life, a cannabis plant will produce more than 400 different chemical compounds. But the presence of just one of those hundreds of compounds has sealed cannabis' fate for nearly a century, making it one of the most persecuted plants on the planet. And all because this one compound happens to interact with the human body in such a way as to produce a complex signature of effects—a "high" unlike any other. Its name is THC. What is THC and what does THC stand for? Tetrahydrocannabinol. More importantly, what does THC do to the brain?

THC is one of the 113 chemical compounds found only in the plant genus Cannabis, which scientists call cannabinoids. THC, however, is unique among all the rest for one, massively important reason: it's the most potently psychoactive.

But exactly what is THC, and why does it produce the wide range of pleasurable (and sometimes not-so-pleasing) effects it does? What does THC do to the brain? How does it affect the body? Is it safe, or as dangerous as heroin, like the federal government says?

Decades of unanswered questions, confusion, and misinformation have distorted the public's understanding of cannabis and the psychoactive cannabinoid that has made it the most popular illicit drug in the world.

I will focus in on the importance of the cannabinoid for recreational and medical users, survey the current research on the drug, and share thoughts about what the future holds for tetrahydrocannabinol.

Let's start with the basics: what is THC and what does THC stand for?

THC is an acronym for the unwieldy and eight-syllable full name of the chemical compound in weed that makes you high. Tetrahydrocannabinol. Its chemical name is (–)-trans-delta 9-tetrahydrocannabinol if you want to get really technical.

The word is imposing at first, but with a little practice, you'll find it rolls off the tongue. Its elegance is in its meter, three trochees followed by an iambic flourish. TE-tra-HY-dro-CAN-na-bin-OL.

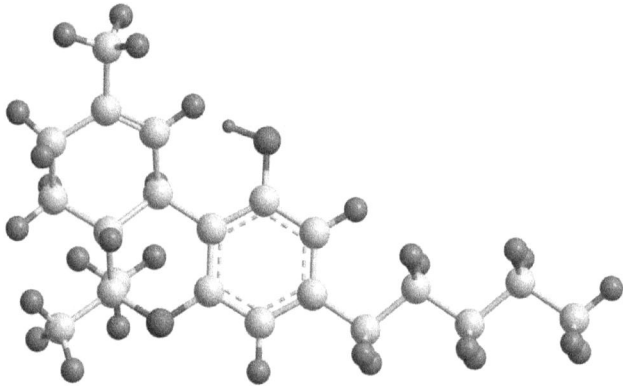

Now that you sound like an expert, let's actually make you into one. Here's your fundamental fact sheet about THC.

delta-9 Tetrahydrocannabinol Is Psychoactive

For most people, psychoactivity is as awesome as it sounds. The word refers to the way THC stimulates or "activates" specific psychological responses generally, but not always, associated with euphoria. In short, THC is psychoactive because it affects the mind.

Of course, the mind and body are connected, and therefore the psychoactive effects of cannabis are both psychological and physiological.

We have the pioneering scientist Dr. Allyn Howlett to thank for making the discovery that showed us why. In 1988, she uncovered where and how THC was attaching to the brain. In short, she discovered the secret link between tetrahydrocannabinol and the human endocannabinoid system (ECS).

THC And The Endocannabinoid System: The Secret To Why You're High

Tetrahydrocannabinol? Endocannabinoid system? Understanding the biochemistry of cannabis definitely requires picking up some new vocabulary. But they're key to understanding what THC is and how it affects us.

In fact, the key makes a good explanatory metaphor. The ECS is like a vast system of locks, or chemical receptors, and keys, the chemicals that bind to them. Some keys only work on a specific lock. Other keys fit in multiple locks. The human body has evolved to produce its own keys, or "endogenous cannabinoids," for those locks.

If you're a runner, you already know all about this. That runner's high you crave is caused by anandamide (the key) binding with cannabinoid receptors (the locks) in your nervous system. Anandamide is THC's endogenous equivalent. Now that's getting high on your own supply!

Amazingly, the cannabinoids the cannabis plant produces happen to bind to those same receptors. They're keys from nature that fit the locks in our ECS. That doesn't mean humans evolved for cannabis, however.

Rather, humans have taken advantage of the fact for enjoyment and health. And we've been doing it for millennia.

What Does THC Do To The Brain?

When you consume cannabis, you introduce its cannabinoids into your body. Once inside, they're metabolized and enter the bloodstream. From there, they bind to receptors CB1 and CB2, which are concentrated in the brain and central nervous system.

Astonishingly, there are 10 times more CB1 receptors in the brain than μ-opioid receptors, which are responsible for the effects of morphine. CB2 receptors hang out exclusively on the cells of the immune system. For that reason, cannabis has significant medicinal applications, in addition to its more popular recreational uses.

So what does THC do to the brain? THC isn't the only cannabinoid that can bind to CB1 and CB2 receptors. But when it does, the ECS stimulates the release of dopamine in the brain, creating a sense of euphoria and relaxation. In short, a high.

How THC Gets You High

CB1 receptors throughout the brain and nervous system modulate movement, memory, cognition, sensory perceptions, and even time perception. According to NIDA, tetrahydrocannabinol "over activates" the functions typically regulated by the ECS, like mood, appetite, cognition, and perception.

Ultimately, it's the sum total of all of these changes that creates the overall sensation we love to call "being high". And it accounts for why everyone's high is unique, and why highs can vary from buzzed to baked to way, way too high. There are just so many factors at play. Changes that feel good to someone might make someone else feel uncomfortable.

Then, there are the more mysterious effects of delta-9-THC on the brain. Remember anandamide, our body's own version of THC? Researchers believe anandamide may have something to do with our brain's ability to forget.

At first glance, this fact seems to confirm the oft-cited concern that cannabis use reduces short-term memory capabilities. Yet the power to forget can be incredibly beneficial for those suffering from traumatic memories, like people with PTSD. Hence the promising findings that tetrahydrocannabinol can treat a range of psychological disorders related to trauma.

What Does Tetrahydrocannabinol Do To The Body?

THC doesn't just bind to receptors in your brain. Their network extends throughout the body. Most of the bodily sensations you experience when you consume cannabis are actually the result of changes in your brain. But cannabinoids can also act on ECS receptors all through the body, creating a range of beneficial effects.

Importantly, there are receptors in the immune system, which is why THC can act as a powerful anti-inflammatory, but can also reduce the immune system's effectiveness.

In the digestive tract, THC can stimulate the release of the "hunger hormone" ghrelin and help ease nausea. A little morsel of cannabis history: despite prohibition, the FDA has approved a synthetic form of THC as an appetite stimulant and an antiemetic for AIDS and chemotherapy patients.

There are even CB2 receptors in our skin. Cannabis topical creams are quickly becoming popular as pain relievers and skincare products. The ability to absorb THC into the skin means people can use the cannabinoid for therapeutic benefits without the psychotropic effects.

The Medicinal Benefits Of Tetrahydrocannabinol

Since THC has become synonymous with marijuana in our everyday lexicon, it can be easy to overlook or discount the medicinal benefits of the cannabinoid. And while it's true that the chemical is highly prized by recreational users, researchers continue to identify innovative ways to use it as a medicine.

Anti-Inflammatory

We've already mentioned how THC affects the body's immune system: it's a powerful anti-inflammatory drug. Inflammation is an underlying factor that contributes to or complicates a wide range of diseases, which means tetrahydrocannabinol has a role to play in treating all of them.

From autoimmune diseases to neuro-degenerative disorders like multiple sclerosis to depression, cannabis has demonstrated its potency as a therapeutic treatment.

Cancer

The potential to use cannabis as part of a cancer treatment is one of the most promising—and most overstated—of THC's benefits. It's far more likely that a physician will prescribe cannabis as a treatment for the harsh side-effects of cancer treatments like chemotherapy and radiation.

However, studies are beginning to identify the "cancer-killing" properties of tetrahydrocannabinol. According to researchers who've investigated the effects of cannabis on tumors in animals, THC can cause cancer cells to eat themselves. The results are incredible: shrunken tumors and a reduction in the prevalence of cancer cells.

Mood Disorders

In addition to helping people with PTSD process and forget traumatic memory associations, tetrahydrocannabinol's short-term effects can improve mood disorders like depression and anxiety. Some have even suggested THC can help people with ADHD.

There is somewhat of a double-edged sword to using THC as a mood disorder treatment, though. Some studies have found that long-term effects of cannabis use can hasten the onset of certain psychological disorders. If you're more prone to schizophrenia or psychosis, regular cannabis use can make you more vulnerable to those symptoms.

Chronic Pain

One of the most popular medical uses for THC is as a pain-reliever. And compared to the dangerous and addictive opioids that are flooding the pharmaceutical market in the United States, cannabis is incredibly safe.

From temporary muscle soreness to constant neuropathic pain, THC's ability to reduce information and stimulate the release of dopamine—just like opioids—make it such a powerful medicine for treating pain and related symptoms.

Sleep Disorders

Inducing euphoria and relaxation, two effects associated with THC's recreational use, are also helpful for treating sleep disorders. Around 1 out of every 3 people experience some form of insomnia. And while prescription sleep aids can help in the short term, they're ineffective and sometimes dangerous with long-term use.

But the old cliche of the "midnight toker" has emerged for exactly this reason. Cannabis relaxes both mind and body. Certain strains, traditionally indicas, have stronger sedative effects than others.

Digestive Disorders

Even the FDA has recognized THC's ability to soothe pain and reduce nausea and other symptoms related to gastrointestinal distress. Thanks to endocannabinoid receptors in the digestive tract, cannabis can help folks suffering from severe GI-tract diseases like Crohn's and irritable bowel syndrome.

This list of the medical benefits of tetrahydrocannabinol is impressive. And as barriers to research crumble, it will only continue to get longer.

THC And Recreational Cannabis Use

Despite its medicinal properties, THC's claim to fame (and infamy) is the euphoric high it produces. Recreational use of marijuana is all about dialing in the perfect ratio of effects for each individual. And the recreational market, especially where it's above ground, continues to develop new and innovative ways of getting high.

Whether it's new strains boasting previous unheard of THC concentrations, new devices for obtaining and consuming cannabis concentrates, or new techniques for produces the highest quality edibles, the recreational market is no doubt one of the most exciting emerging horizons in the cannabis industry worldwide.

At the moment, no trend dominates the recreational cannabis scene more than concentrates. So what is THC concentrate?

THC Concentrates And The Brave New World Of

Dabbing

There are a few methods for extracting cannabinoids from the herbaceous matter of dried cannabis flowers. Some are safer than others. But the objective for each of them is the same: extract the maximum amount of cannabinoids and terpenes from the cannabis plant.

Butane, CO_2 and alcohol extraction methods each have their own merits. And each is able to produce cannabis concentrates with THC concentration levels around 90 percent or higher. Compare that to the average of 25-30 percent THC boasted by the most potent cannabis strains, and you can see why concentrates have become so popular among recreational users.

In final form, concentrates are rich and flavorful substances with an amber color and sticky, gooey texture. They can be consumed purely, or mixed with edible waxes, oils and tinctures in the forms of beverages and tasty treats.

One method of consuming concentrates, however, has catapulted to popularity among recreational users: dabbing. Dabbing is the process of super-heating a glass or metallic element, placing a dab of concentrate on it, and inhaling the ensuing vapors.

Concentrate extraction removes all the bitter plant matter from the cannabis. Yet it maintains the presence of the plant terpenes that give cannabis its taste and smell. Hence, the experience of dabbing, or inhaling the vapor of sublimated concentrates, provides incomparably rich flavors compared to just smoking flowers.

Cannabis Strains With The Highest Concentration Of Tetrahydrocannabinol

Dabbing affords recreational users a massive dose of tetrahydrocannabinol, far greater than any herbaceous cannabis could provide. In other words, dabbing will make you higher than you ever thought possible, and certainly higher than you could get otherwise.

Yet for some, inhaling vapors with upwards of 90 percent tetrahydrocannabinol creates too strong of an effect. This can tip the euphoria of a good high into the anxiousness of a bad one. In that case, recreational users seek out strains with high THC concentrations. Here are some of the most potent THC-dominant strains around.

- Godfather OG // Indica // 34.04 percent THC
- Super Glue // Hybrid // 32.14 percent THC
- Strawberry Banana // Hybrid // 31.62 percent THC
- Venom OG Kush // Indica // 31.04 percent THC

As you may have noticed, the prevalence of the "OG" moniker reveals that these "ocean grown" strains hail from the California region. With an ideal climate and the most established breeding and cultivation programs, the strongest cannabis strains in the world come from sunny CA.

Fire It Up! Why You Need Heat To Enjoy THC

Since we've taken a good look at the recreational dimensions of tetrahydrocannabinol, now's a good time to mention a very important fact about consuming THC.

In it's "raw form," tetrahydrocannabinol is totally inert and will do nothing for you. Again, the form in which tetrahydrocannabinol manifests in cannabis plants is inactive. If you ate a handful of dried cannabis flowers, you wouldn't get high. But you would have a stomach ache trying to digest the plant fibers! You need heat to make tetrahydrocannabinol work.

So what does THC do when you apply heat to it

Technically speaking, the cannabinoid that appears in cannabis is THCA. The "A" designates its acidic form. It takes heat to convert THCA to the psychoactive delta-9 tetrahydrocannabinol. That's why you have to apply a flame to dried cannabis. Not just to combust the buds to produce smoke to inhale, but to actually activate the THC.

That activation process is called decarboxylation, or "decarb" for short. Decarbing your cannabis is an absolutely indispensable step when making edibles. Without it, you're just eating a bunch of raw THCA.

But heating THC to the point of decarboxylation is challenging. It's too easy to apply too much heat, which results in boiling off the tetrahydrocannabinol completely. Not good!

What The Future Holds For THC

While breeders continue to craft strains with record-breaking tetrahydrocannabinol concentrations, THC's future is undeniably in the realm of concentrates.

In fact, one of the most important realizations to come out of dabbing culture has profound implications for the future of cannabis in general. The "entourage effect" refers to the synergistic interactions between tetrahydrocannabinol, terpenes, and other cannabinoids. Concentrate production keeps these compounds intact. And that means you don't just inhale pure THC vapor, but vapor consisting of all of those chemicals combined.

One thing we know is that on its own, THC's effects are is kind of a "directionless." There's no way to determine where, how, or how much it will interact with various parts of the ECS.

It seems that terpenes, however, which are basically the plants' essential oils, aren't just there for smell and taste. They also seem to act as guard rails, allowing users to "steer" THC into different chemical pathways and thus, produce different effects.

Knowledge about these interactions is still in its infancy. But recreational users, not researchers, are paving the way by experimenting with different terpene profiles and cannabinoid concentrations. And the demand they're causing for concentrates is responsible for many of the recent innovations in extraction and vaping techniques.

CBD vs. THC: The Difference Between The Two Cannabinoids

Having knowledge about the key differences between CBD and THC is super important for finding the right cannabis products and understanding how they'll affect you.

THC and CBD are the most well-known and sought-after chemicals produced by the cannabis plant. But in the battle of CBD vs THC, who comes out on top? Is it the legendary THC, producer of wonderful sensations and euphoric elation? Or will it be CBD, the newcomer surging in popularity due to its wide-ranging health and wellness benefits? What are the differences between the two cannabinoids? And is framing it as a contest— as THC vs CBD —the best way to think about those differences?

As cannabis markets expand, consumers have more choice than ever. And one of the most important choices cannabis consumers have to make is how much THC and CBD they want their products to contain.

Knowing the differences between CBD and THC is essential for making mindful, intentional choices in the dispensary. Understanding how they work together can help you create cannabis experiences that best meet your needs and desires.

CBD: Knowing what it really is

First, CBD is non-psychoactive. In other words, it won't make you feel high. This point is crucial because it makes CBD derived from hemp available in some places where marijuana is prohibited. However, hemp-derived CBD is still not technically legal in all 50 states under federal law.

Second, CBD is responsible for many of the significant medical and therapeutic benefits of cannabis. And that's why you'll always hear people talking about CBD products when they're using cannabis for health and wellness.

THC: A Very Short Introduction

Even non-consumers of cannabis have heard about THC. Tetrahydrocannabinol, a.k.a. THC, is the chemical that produces the euphoric, stimulating sensations from cannabis use we call being "high."

THC isn't the only cannabinoid that produces those effects, but it is the only one that exists in significant enough quantities in cannabis products to get a consumer high. For this reason, THC is the ine qua non of recreational cannabis use.

But that's not to say there aren't medical or therapeutic uses for THC. In fact, the mostly cognitive and psychological effects of THC on the human body, including pleasing alterations in mood, perception and thought, have a wide range of medicinal applications.

CBD vs THC: The Major Differences for Recreational Consumers

Now you know about CBD and THC in a nutshell. And since we're simplifying things, here are the two most important points of difference between the cannabinoids.

CBD doesn't produce a high, while THC will definitely get you high.

Medical, health, and wellness users tend to put an emphasis on CBD, while recreational consumers tend to favor THC.

It's important to stress that those neat divisions are only useful as a quick point of reference. The reality is that there are plenty of reasons for recreational consumers to want products with CBD. Just as there are many medicinal benefits to THC.

So, let's dive deeper into the question of THC vs CBD. Beyond the simple difference that THC will get you high and CBD won't, what are the key differences between the two for recreational consumers?

CBD vs THC: Emotional And Mental Effects

For most cannabis consumers, THC produces a palette of pleasing sensations that include euphoria, sensory stimulation, positive mood alterations and even feelings of improved cognition. Generally, these experiences aren't overwhelming. But sometimes they can be, tipping into anxiety and paranoia.

CBD doesn't produce any mental and emotional effects of its own. But it absolutely influences how THC creates those effects. For recreational users, CBD can act as a counterweight to balance and level out a strong reaction to THC.

Of course, the opposite is also true. For people who crave the sensations of THC and want nothing to stand in their way, eliminating CBD can effectively make a product more potent. That's the point behind THC concentrates.

THC vs. CBD: Physical Effects and Therapeutic Benefits

CBD Hemp Oil - A Scientific Guide For Cbd Use And Pain Relief

Recreational users who prefer a more body-focused high can benefit from cannabis products containing CBD. Cannabidiol has a calming effect on the body. It reduces inflammation and helps treat pain by blocking pain receptors.

These mellowed, relaxed bodily sensations can help round out a cerebral high for a more whole-body experience. The physical effects and therapeutic benefits of CBD can even highlight and emphasize the pleasurable effects THC has on your body in the first place.

THC vs. CBD: The Key Differences for Medical Cannabis Users

For medical cannabis users, the differences between THC and CBD are very important. Both cannabinoids offer therapeutic and medicinal benefits. But CBD offers them without psychoactive side effects. For that reason, CBD is ideal for patients who do not desire the effects of THC or who cannot as safely consume THC, like children.

Indeed, CBD is so well-researched for medical applications because of the fact that it doesn't produce the effects of a high. In many places, that's enough to make CBD products legal, as long as they don't contain THC above a certain threshold.

CBD vs. THC: Health Benefits

In terms of their health benefits, one of the main differences between THC and CBD is the parts of the body that they affect. The endocannabinoid receptors in our body that bind with CBD are distributed throughout the nervous system and concentrated in the spleen. THC receptors, on the other hand, are concentrated in the brain.

CBD, therefore, produces strong anti-inflammatory effects on the body. And that's good for a number of health reasons. Many diseases involve or are worsened by inflammation, so reducing it can help treat those diseases.

But CBD goes one step further. It can also protect cells, especially nerve cells, from damage and deterioration due to inflammation. This makes CBD a possibly effective treatment for seizures, epilepsy, MS, and arthritis. Some studies have shown that CBD can stop the spread of cancer cells and in some cases, shrink tumors.

THC vs. CBD: Treatable Symptoms

THC, like CBD, also has anti-inflammatory properties. This makes it great for treating pain, one of the most commonly recommended uses for THC. But because THC receptors are concentrated in the brain, many of the health benefits of the cannabinoid stem from the chemicals it releases there.

Often, medical cannabis users consume THC in order to produce the same effects sought after by recreational consumers. But in the medical context, those effects can actually help treat many of the complicating symptoms associated with severe diseases.

For example, THC can reduce the nausea and vomiting associated with chemotherapy treatments. It can stimulate appetite in people losing weight due to illness or treatments for the illness.

And importantly, THC can help treat mental and cognitive problems associated with illness. Often, severe and chronic diseases cause anxiety and depression, which THC's euphoric effects can help remedy. Indeed, a recent study on THC and Alzheimer's patients found that the cannabinoid can reduce agitation and other mood disorders in people with dementia.

CBD vs. THC? More Like CBD Plus THC

To conclude this guide to the major differences between CBD and

THC, we should address the elephant in the room. That little "vs." standing between THC vs. CBD.

That "vs." or versus, implies conflict, a winner-take-all battle between the two most prominent cannabinoids. While CBD and THC compliment some of each other's effects, that's not the result of two warring chemicals—it is the result of their working together.

In the same way that CBD can balance a strong THC high and alleviate some of the perceived negative effects of THC, some of the effects of CBD are more potent if the cannabinoid is consumed with THC.

This cooperative relationship between cannabinoids is called the "entourage effect" or "ensemble effect." It's based on the principle that the cannabinoids in cannabis reach their full potential when they operate in concert.

CBD vs. THC: Crafting Your Ideal Cannabis Experience

The differences between CBD and THC are real, and they make all the difference in your cannabis experience. So whether you like to think about it as CBD vs THC, or THC vs CBD, now that you know a little bit about what makes them unique, you can make more mindful, intentional choices about the cannabis products you use, while feeling confident that those products will produce the effect you want.

Matthew Stone

CBD Success Stories

How can one plant compound help with so many ailments?

The CBD success stories we've heard about CBD oil have astounded us. Here are six people with chronic pain and/or a crippling disease who have experienced relief from this high-end CBD oil.

CBD is a plant compound that has shown to help with mental clarity, productivity, and peace of mind, a stronger immune system, pain relief, and so much more. The research supporting CBD's many positive factors is piling high, and a recent study shows that people tend to drop their traditional medicine once they experience the benefits. It's seemingly a veritable wonder 'drug.' Given the feedback we've heard firsthand, the only thing that's leaves you wondering about CBD hemp oil is the stupefying fact that the powers that be are trying to keep it from being readily available to the public.

While medical marijuana legality is still under question, CBD hemp oil from industrialized hemp is a safe, legal go-to. Unless of course, you ask the DEA. Cannabinoidal (CBD) is the non-psychoactive compound found in both hemp and marijuana that is responsible for communicating with our own endocannabinoid system, which in turn promotes many health benefits. All sorts of people with various ailments, from athletes to senior citizens, are reporting transformational CBD success stories.

The internet is flooded with CBD brands. But the quality and source of the herb, the extraction method used, and the bioavailability of the compound are some crucial factors that affect the healing potential of your CBD. Many users have tried other brands and came back to Superior CBD again for its unparalleled efficacy.

Let's take a look at these six accounts from people, all across the USA, who are reporting CBD success stories with Superior CBD.

Extreme Sports & Leviticus

Eric Lakey, Georgia, Chronic pain & kidney cancer

Eric lived up his twenties riding dirt bikes, motorbikes, water skiing, skiing and engaging in other high-thrill sports. But, like many extreme sports enthusiasts, Eric got beat up — a lot. He injured his posterior knee on his right leg and had to go in for surgery and take pain killers for a short while. In his 30s, Eric suffered a compound fracture and broke the left ankle. A few years later he broke some ribs. With each injury, he took pain meds, but he never got addicted to them.

In his 40s, Eric started suffering from major back problems. He went in for an MRI, which showed he had seven bad disks from his neck down to his spine. A pain clinic performed Radiofrequency ablation on him, a procedure that involves burning his nerves. They also put him on extensive painkillers: four doses of oratab (opiates) which is hydrocodone and 10mg/500mg acetaminophen. He took this concoction for eight years straight before switching to four doses of hydrocodone bitartrate, 7.5mg 325mg acetaminophen per day. Such a heavy dose of opioids is often linked to negative side effects, such as Opioid-induced bowel dysfunction (OIBD), with all sorts of gastrointestinal issues.

The opiods enabled him to continue working as a commercial/industrial electrician, by managing the pain. But the more he went to the pain clinic, the more he got turned off by the people. "They were just trying to make money, like the people who run the pharmaceuticals." Eric could tell they didn't really care about him and his well-being. Instead, he felt they were just trying to push the painkillers that the pharmaceuticals sold.

In November 2016, Eric decided he wanted to try to get off

painkillers, while he was on a vacation. A friend got him a THC concentrate, which he vaped. "The THC helped with the opioid withdrawal symptoms, but not with the pain. That's when I started doing research on CBD. I looked it up online and the first thing I found was Superior CBD Oil from Honey Colony. And I just had a sense I had to get that CBD — no other brand."

He started taking Superior CBD this past February. Eric is now in his late 50s. The week before he received the delivery, Eric got the flu. A trip to the doctor revealed he had he had a four-centimeter tumor in one of his kidneys and the vein going into it was twice the size it should've been.

Eric's not entirely sure what the full diagnosis of the tumor is, but he says, "It's been a roller coaster, but honestly, CBD oil makes me feel fantastic. I don't feel the kidney pain at all. I feel great."

His joint and muscle pain also was severely reduced with the Superior CBD oil — so much so that he weaned himself down from four to only one and a half pills a day. He would take himself totally off it, but he's trying to healthily cut back since coming off opioids too quickly might mess with his serotonin levels.

Although it's only been a short time since Eric's began taking CBD, he's reaping numerous health benefits. Eric started out with a morning dose of 10 drops of CBD a day, but now he takes 12-14 drops, three times a day. "In the past week, I noticed that a scar I had on my face from a motorcycle accident I'd had in my 20s has totally disappeared."

The possibility of scars healing through CBD seemed strange, even to us. But Elizabeth Moriarty, Superior's formulator, shed some light on the issue:

"Scar tissue is in essence fundamentally similar to fibrosis in its constitution, and there are studies aplenty showing that CBD reduces fibrosis. So, yes, I consider it possible (for CBD to heal scars). Research and discovery of the endocannabinoid system and its integrated influences and involvement in body systems are so very young. As much as we are seeing a new study every day, we are in the baby days of learning."

Eric is taking small steps to improve his health in other ways, as well. He started eating according to the laws of the Old Testament, in Leviticus, and drinks nothing but water. "Everything on this earth is here to heal us. We have so much poison from all the toxins. I'm not where I should be with my health, but I'm a lot better than I was."

War & Peace

Glenn, Army Retiree, Maryland, Diabetes, anxiety, PTSD

Glenn, who spent the majority of his adult life serving as a pilot and logistician in the U.S. Army, suffers from diabetes, edema in his extremities, anxiety, hypertension and high blood pressure — not to mention PTSD from combat deployments. "I had a challenge with stress and flare ups with my kids and spouse. It usually happens around people I know, because I feel more comfortable to let out all the stress." Glenn has a large family with several children and grandchildren, so his house is often very busy.

"I was about 50 when I retired from the military. I couldn't complain while I was still active, but when I got off, I told them about my chronic conditions and they gave me all sorts of drugs. I was taking 5-7 drugs: one for blood pressure, another for anxiety, another for diabetes, and more for edema, anxiety, etc. I took them for short while and felt they were just masking the issues and not really healing me. I expected the miracle cure from taking the right drugs but that's not what they do."

Glenn and his family only became aware of holistic alternatives when his wife decided to make their kitchen food-coloring free. "That afternoon we could see the difference in my daughter, a smart, lively girl who was diagnosed with ADHD. So then, my wife took out all preservatives from the kitchen, and she started cooking own bread and all that. Then we got on the train with essential oils. Next, my wife decided to try 40 days of a sugar-free, gluten-free lifestyle, and she got rid of headaches, acne and other issues."

That's when Glenn started looking into CBD for his health issues. He said "to heck with all the pharmaceuticals" and put his bag of drugs under the sink."That's when I started reading about Superior CBD. Superior CBD seemed like a real high-quality supplement, so I decided to give Superior a try, despite the fact there are many other vendors.

"I take 5-8 drops of CBD oil, and within no more than a few minutes I feel a lot more at ease with myself and others around me. I used to have to leave the room whenever my grandchildren were over because the extra commotion raised the ante and made me more anxious — and now i can put up with more anxiety and stress. I can actually enjoy the situation and the time with my family.

"It's a natural cure. It has relieved my PTSD issues, swelling, and some of the diabetes effects I was suffering from. It puts me at ease, and it gives me a deep sense of peace."

Pain Meds Be Gone

Daphne Herbst, Wisconsin, Chronic Back pain and loss of appetite

Daphne, a 70-year old retiree, has been suffering from chronic back pain for 15 years. Due to the pain, she lost her appetite. "It's really hard when you're just looking at food and you want to eat it but you can't. You're losing weight and getting weak, but there is just nothing you can do."

Daphne was on Fentanyl patches for her back, which is an opioid with side effects that included gastrointestinal issues, lightheadedness, dizziness, headaches, and more. Often, when she experiences acute pain, doctors put her on "breakthrough medication," which is the application of an opioid, 5 to 20 percent of the dose patients usually take to manage their pain that goes to work quickly and lasts for a short period of time. "I was taking those things for so long that my body was just used to them."

Faced with the reality that her meds no longer provided her with the relief, Daphne got her first delivery of Superior CBD in July 2017. "Originally I started with six drops, twice a day. Then, I switched to six drops, once a day. I noticed the same effect. It gave me an appetite, and it also gives me a sense of better well-being. With less pain and more energy from the food, I'm more productive."

When Superior CBD oil wasn't available for a few months due to the politics involving CBD, Daphne tried using another brand of CBD. "It wasn't nearly effective. I was so happy I could start ordering again."

Getting To the Land Of Zzzzzzs

Lisa Miller, California, Broken neck and open dislocation in her ankle

When Lisa was 19, she suffered a broken neck from a terrible car accident. She's been suffering chronic neck pain ever since. What's more, when she was in her 40s, Lisa dislocated her foot and currently has an open dislocation (a joint displacement accompanied by a break in the skin) in her ankle. "I wasn't sleeping at all — the pain was so bad." As a nurse, sleep-deprivation made long shifts in the hospital agonizing.

Two years ago, in her late 50s, Lisa heard about CBD oil from a friend. Lisa ordered Brown Botanical's CBD. "I didn't notice much of a difference in my symptoms with that CBD. So, after awhile, I decided to look into something else."

A friend told her about Honey Colony and how they are a trustworthy health site. So two years ago Lisa went online and started ordering Superior CBD. "I noticed a huge difference between it and the CBD I'd tried earlier. I like the fact that there are no additives and it's very clean."

Lisa has been taking 20 drops of Superior CBD in the morning, twice a day. "It's been life-changing. It helps me sleep — I can sleep through the night now. It also helps ease my pain by relaxing and releasing my muscles. It also changes my mood, both energetically and emotionally. Sometimes i can get kind of anxious, and it really helps with that, too.

"I just went away for four days and forgot to take my CBD with me, and I did not sleep well at all."

Chemo & Cancer

Beverly Schwarz, Chicago, Bladder cancer

In 2013, Beverly, a resilient 75-year old woman, was diagnosed with stage three bladder cancer. The doctors put her on a ton of antibiotics, and didn't give her much hope. "They put me on chemo for seven months — that's a lot of chemo. After that, my bladder didn't work anymore. But, I'm still around."

Her daughter told Beverly about Superior CBD over a year ago. "It really builds up your immune system. It makes you feel better and more energized. It also helps with the pain, and it calms me down a little bit."

Since she's been taking it, Beverly's been very active. "The doctors saw me and said, 'Keep on doing what you're doing.' They didn't expect to still see me around."

Beverly also takes turmeric and other holistic herbs. "I think Honey Colony has a really good product. When Superior CBD wasn't around for a few months, I tried other CBD brands, but the healing effects just weren't the same."

An Enhanced Quality of Life

With 10X bio-availability and fast-absorption, Superior is continuing to report inspiring CBD success stories. Not only was it designed to help relieve many chronic conditions, but it also balances the nervous and musculoskeletal system. This special formulation synergizes hemp oil with other medicinal herbs used in ancient medicine.

The fact it falls under all legal parameters for a safe drug, Honey Colony has been seemingly targeted for selling it. Moriarty shared her thoughts on the politics of CBD:

"There are some very serious business challenges faced by companies that produce and sell hemp-derived CBD products. The public confusion about the legal status of these products is understandable, given the fact that both hemp and marijuana are cannabis species.More significantly, perplexing statements and introduced legislation by politicians is likely due to a combination of befuddlement — in the face of many moving parts of a complex industry — and hidden political agendas."

There's a battle underway, between those who are committed to maintaining public access to hemp-derived CBD (as well as other minor cannabinoids) as a vital plant nutrient, and those who are equally committed to pharmaceuticalizing isolated compounds within the plant and gaining patent rights and exclusivity of access through the institutional medical complex.

Due to the political confusion surrounding the status of hemp-derived CBD, financial institutions are wary of involvement with companies that produce and sell CBD products — and perhaps, those invested in financial industries are also well-invested in the pharmaceutical and medical industries.

Selling CBD is a tough business, but Honey Colony is dedicated to overcoming the challenges and getting Superior to those who need it.

1. Rick Simpson

Rick Simpson is known for inventing hemp-oil medicine that he claims treated his own skin cancer after he was a 'chemical zombie' from all the drugs he had taken as a cancer sufferer. After curing himself and hundreds of others with his cannabis oil, Rick tried to take his medicine to Canadian authorities. However, the move backfired and the authorities tried to prosecute him. Today, Rick is considered a hero in the medical marijuana world with a huge following of believers. Watch his documentary, 'Run From The Cure' and see for yourself.

2. Shona Banda

A sufferer of Crohn's Disease for eight years, Shona was bedridden and could only walk with a cane. Diagnosed as terminally ill, Shona decided to explore alternative remedies in a last bid to save her life. Shona saw Rick Simpson's video and began to treat herself with cannabis oil and voila! She is now considered cured and has a normal life. She subsequently wrote a book, 'Live Free or Die,' detailing the weed experience that saved her life.

3. Charlotte Figi

Six-year-old Charlotte is the miniature miracle who suffered from an untreatable form of epilepsy and used medical marijuana to cure herself. By the time she was two years old her parents had literally tried all medications to cure her – some which nearly ended in her demise. Enduring some 50 seizures a night, her parents managed to get her a medical marijuana card in Colorado. After her first dose of high CBD oil her seizures immediately stopped, her parents claim. She emerged out of her catatonic state and her parents got to meet her for the first time. Charlotte has since featured on a CNN documentary, documenting her miraculous story.

4. Kristen Courtney

Juicing raw cannabis is the Crohn's Disease health cure that Kristen claims saved her life. Diagnosed at 16 with juvenile rheumatoid arthritis, the illness quickly turned into an auto immune disorder that left her bedridden for four years. Finally, the teen and her mother began to look for alternative treatments. Kristen began juicing raw cannabis, and after a month she claims her pain stopped and her recovery began. She is now an advocate for medical marijuana treatment for fellow sufferers.

5. Peter Germain

Peter suffered from type 2 diabetes, which he says impacted on his quality of life on a daily basis. After being introduced to cannabis oil, he began to see results within just six weeks. His blood sugar levels reduced considerably, and he lost 50 pounds. Today, Peter claims digesting cannabis oil cured his diabetes and obesity.

6. David Triplett

David claims to have cured himself of two cancerous lesions using cannabis oil from his dispensary. He initially received a prescription chemo cream, but David decided not to apply the treatment after seeing disturbing images of people who had used it. Instead, he began treating the lesions with cannabis ointment which, after three to four weeks of application, removed the cancer.

7. Cheryl Shuman

After being diagnosed with cancer, Beverly Hills celebrity Cheryl Shuman began taking a cocktail of medications and up to 27 morphine tablets a day in a bid to overcome the disease. However, after learning about cannabis oil, Cheryl started to treat herself. She says the treatment cured her in 90 days and remains in remission to this day.

8. Dennis Hill

"Cannabis kills cancer!" That is the message often repeated by biochemist Dennis Hill, who claims to have treated his own cancer using Rick Simpson's cannabis concentrate. After a three-month stint, in which Hill combined healthy eating and exercise with cannabis doses, he says his tumor disappeared. After six months, Hill says he rid his body of cancer for good.

If there weren't already enough good reasons to legalize pot, the discovery that marijuana may have the medical potential to cure people from debilitating illnesses, as the inspirational stories suggest, may prove to be the most convincing argument yet. Weed Geek reveals the heart-felt triumphs of those who claim medical marijuana miraculously saved their lives.

REFERENCES

Borgelt LM, Franson KL, Nussbaum AM, Wang GS (February 2013). "The pharmacologic and clinical effects of medical cannabis" (Submitted manuscript). Pharmacotherapy (Review). 33 (2): 195–209. doi:10.1002/phar.1187. PMID 23386598.

"Sativex (Cannabidiol/Tetrahydrocannabinol) Bayer Label" (PDF). bayer.ca. Retrieved 28 June 2018.

"Epidiolex (Cannabidiol) FDA Label" (PDF). fda.gov. Retrieved 28 June 2018.

Mechoulam R, Parker LA, Gallily R (November 2002). "Cannabidiol: an overview of some pharmacological aspects". Journal of Clinical Pharmacology. 42 (11 Suppl): 11S–19S. doi:10.1002/j.1552-4604.2002.tb05998.x. PMID 12412831.

Scuderi C, Filippis DD, Iuvone T, Blasio A, Steardo A, Esposito G (May 2009). "Cannabidiol in medicine: a review of its therapeutic potential in CNS disorders". Phytotherapy Research (Review). 23 (5): 597–602. doi:10.1002/ptr.2625. PMID 18844286.

R. F. Keeler (30 November 1983). Handbook of Natural Toxins. CRC Press. p. 477. ISBN 978-0-8247-1893-0.

Pisanti S, Malfitano AM, Ciaglia E, Lamberti A, Ranieri R, Cuomo G, Abate M, Faggiana G, Proto MC, Fiore D, Laezza C, Bifulco M (July 2017). "Cannabidiol: State of the art and new challenges for therapeutic applications". Pharmacol. Ther. 175: 133–150. doi:10.1016/j.pharmthera.2017.02.041. PMID 28232276.

Campos AC, Moreira FA, Gomes FV, Del Bel EA, Guimarães FS (December 2012). "Multiple mechanisms involved in the large-spectrum therapeutic potential of cannabidiol in psychiatric disorders". Philosophical Transactions of the Royal Society of London. Series B, Biological Sciences (Review). 367 (1607): 3364–78. doi:10.1098/rstb.2011.0389. PMC 3481531 . PMID 23108553.

Aizpurua-Olaizola O, Soydaner U, Öztürk E, Schibano D, Simsir Y, Navarro P, Etxebarria N, Usobiaga A (February 2016). "Evolution of the Cannabinoid and Terpene Content during the Growth of Cannabis sativa Plants from Different Chemotypes". Journal of Natural Products. 79 (2): 324–31. doi:10.1021/acs.jnatprod.5b00949. PMID 26836472.

Iseger TA, Bossong MG (March 2015). "A systematic review of the antipsychotic properties of cannabidiol in humans". Schizophrenia Research. 162 (1–3): 153–61. doi:10.1016/j.schres.2015.01.033. PMID 25667194.

Bergamaschi, M. M., Queiroz, R. H. C., Chagas, M. H. N, de Oliveira, D. C. G., De Martinis, B. S., ... Crippa, J. A. S. (2011, May). Cannabidiol reduces the anxiety induced by simulated public speaking in treatment-naïve social phobia patients. Neuropsychopharmacology, 36(6), 1219-1226.

Campos, A. C., de Paula Soares, V., Carvalho, M. C., Ferreira, F. R., Vicente, M. A., ... Guimaraes, F. S. (2013, March). Involvement of serotonin-mediated neurotransmission in the dorsal periaqueductal gray matter on cannabidiol chronic effects in panic-like responses in rats [Abstract]. Psychopharmacology, 226(1), 13-24

Cannabis and cannabinoids. (2016, May 27)

cancer.gov/about-cancer/treatment/cam/patient/cannabis-pdq

Devinsky, O., Marsh, E., Friedman, D., Thiele, E., Laux, L., ... Cilio, M. R. (2016, March). Cannabidiol in patients with treatment-resistant epilepsy: an open-label interventional trial [Asbstract]. The Lancet, 15(3), 270-278

thelancet.com/journals/laneur/article/PIIS1474-4422(15)00379-

8/abstract

Olah, A., Toth, B. I, Borbiro, I., Sugawara, K., Szollosi, A. G., ... Biro, T. (2014, July 25). Cannabidiol exerts sebostatic and anti-inflammatory effects on human sebocytes. Journal of Clinical Investigation, 124(9), 3713-3724

jci.org/articles/view/64628

Volkow, N.D. (2015, June 24). The biology and potential therapeutic effects of cannabidiol

drugabuse.gov/about-nida/legislative-activities/testimony-to-congress/2016/biology-potential-therapeutic-effects-cannabidiol

Zias J., Stark H., Sellgman J., et al. Early medical use of cannabis. Nature. 1993;363:215. [PubMed]

Schlesinger S. Untersuchung der Cannabis sativa. Repertorium fur die Pharmacie. 1840:190–208.

Decourtive E. Note sur le haschisch. CR Hebd Séances Acad Sci. 1848;26:509–510.

Mechoulam R. Cannabinoid chemistry. In: Mechoulam R, ed. Marijuana. New York, NY; London, UK: Academic Press. 1973:1–99.

Mechoulam R., Hanus L. A historical overview of chemical research on cannabinoids. Chem Phys Lipids. 2000;108:1–13. [PubMed]

Gaoni Y., Mechoulam R. Isolation, structure and partial synthesis of the active constituent of hashish. J Am Chem Soc. 1964;86:1646–1647.

Waller CW. JJ., Buelke J., Turner CE. Marihuana, an annotated bibliography. Res Inst Pharmacy Sci Univ Mississippi. 1976 and yearly updates.

Fraser JD. Withdrawal symptoms in cannabis indica addicts. Lancet. 1949;2:747. [PubMed]

Grinspoon L., Bakalar JB., Zimmer L., Morgan JP. Marijuana

addiction. Science. 1997;277:749–author reply 750-742. [PubMed]

Kaymakcalan S. The addictive potential of cannabis. Bull Narc. 1981;33:21–31. [PubMed]

Jones RT., Benowitz N., Bachman J. Clinical studies of cannabis tolerance and dependence. Ann N Y Acad Sci. 1976;282:221–239. [PubMed]

Nordstrom BR., Levin FR. Treatment of cannabis use disorders: a review of the literature. Am J Addict. 2007;16:331–342. [PubMed]

Bernoussi A., Brandibas G. Cannabis addiction and Telic Dominance Scale. Encephale. 2003;29:519–526. [PubMed]

Budney AJ., Moore BA., Rocha HL., Higgins ST. Clinical trial of abstinencebased vouchers and cognitive-behavioral therapy for cannabis dependence. J Consult Clin Psychol. 2006;74:307–316. [PubMed]

Gardner EL. Addictive potential of cannabinoids: the underlying neurobiology. Chem Phys Lipids. 2002;121:267–290. [PubMed]

Maldonado R., Rodriguez de Fonseca F. Cannabinoid addiction: behavioral models and neural correlates. J Neurosci. 2002;22:3326–3331. [PubMed]

Mansbach RS., Nicholson KL., Martin BR., Balster RL. Failure of Delta(9)-tetrahydrocannabinol and CP 55,940 to maintain intravenous self-administration under a fixed-interval schedule in rhesus monkeys. Behav Pharmacol. 1994;5:219–225. [PubMed]

Colombo G., Serra S., Vacca G., Carai MA., Gessa GL. Endocannabinoid system and alcohol addiction: pharmacological studies. Pharmacol Biochem Behav. 2005;81:369–380. [PubMed]

Wang L., Liu J., Harvey-White J., Zimmer A., Kunos G. Endocannabinoid signaling via cannabinoid receptor 1 is involved in ethanol preference and its age-dependent decline in mice. Proc Natl

Acad Sci U S A. 2003;100:1393–1398. [PMC free article] [PubMed]

Cohen C., Perrault G., Voltz C., Steinberg R., Soubrie P. SR141716, a central cannabinoid (CB(1)) receptor antagonist, blocks the motivational and dopaminereleasing effects of nicotine in rats. Behav Pharmacol. 2002;13:451–463. [PubMed]

Miller NS., Gold MS., Klahr AL. The diagnosis of alcohol and cannabis dependence (addiction) in cocaine dependence (addiction). Int J Addict. 1990;25:735–744. [PubMed]

Foltin RW., Fischman MW., Pippen PA., Kelly TH. Behavioral effects of cocaine alone and in combination with ethanol or marijuana in humans. Drug Alcohol Depend. 1993;32:93–106. [PubMed]

Lukas SE., Sholar M., Kouri E., Fukuzako H., Mendelson JH. Marihuana smoking increases plasma cocaine levels and subjective reports of euphoria in male volunteers. Pharmacol Biochem Behav. 1994;48:715–721. [PubMed]

ABOUT THE AUTHOR

Matthew Stone owns a bachelor degree in chemistry from the University of Edinburgh and he took the decision to mix his passion for writing with the one for Chemistry. Over the last year, the author specialized in medical cannabis and published books on CBD, its healing features and the potentials of a cannabinoid that can treat naturally a number of diseases without making use of medicinal products.

www.ingramcontent.com/pod-product-compliance
Lightning Source LLC
Chambersburg PA
CBHW071106240526
45469CB00006BD/2352